A GUIDE TO HEALTHY HORMONES

SECRETS TO BREAST HEALTH

CINDY SIMMONS, HOMEOPATH

A GUIDE TO HEALTHY HORMONES

SECRETS TO BREAST HEALTH

Author: Cindy Simmons

Published by Cindy Simmons at CreateSpace

Copyrights: 2013 Cindy Simmons. All rights reserved

Cover designed by Earl Friedberg www.earlf.com

Editing by Lisa Syed MEd, BEd/TESL, BA lisa@inter-ic.com

ISBN# 978-1484058251

NOTE TO READER:

The information and advice provided in this book are not intended as a substitution for the advice of your physician or healthcare professionals. Consult your physician and healthcare professionals for all issues which may require medical attention or diagnosis, including before administering or undertaking any course of treatment or diet. Neither the author nor the publisher shall be liable or responsible for any loss or damage allegedly arising from any information or suggestion in this book, nor for websites or their content that are referred to in this book.

DISCLAIMER:

All content of this book is based upon research conducted by the author, unless otherwise noted. The author presents this information for educational purposes only. We are not making an attempt to prescribe any medical treatment, and the information contained herein is not intended to replace advice from a medical doctor or qualified health care professional. The author encourages you, however, to make your own health care decisions based upon your research. You are the one responsible for your health and body. The statements, information, products, and service resources in this book are not intended to diagnose, treat, or cure any disease.

ABOUT THE AUTHOR

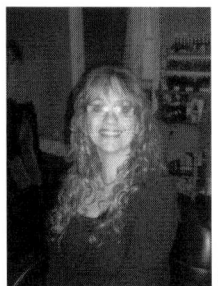 Cindy Simmons is a Natural Medicine Practitioner and Homeopath, and what that means is that she uses natural remedies to treat the whole person. It is her desire to educate people about natural health care and preventative alternatives to teach how the body can heal itself, placing people in the position of true "Informed Consent".

For more than 15 years, Cindy worked as a consultant in the field of Pharmaceutical Clinical Research before going through some life changes and returning to college to study Homeopathic Medicine. As a busy mom with three children of her own and a stepmother to four others, she knew she had to find answers and change the way she was living.

Today, Cindy is the owner of a Natural Medicine Clinic and a Thermography franchise, where she offers women pain-free technology to detect abnormalities in breast tissue in its earliest stages, with zero radiation. In addition to this, she offers homeopathy, nutritional counseling, supplement profiling, and counseling to her clients. She is a Certified Healthy Breast Program Educator. Cindy puts her philosophies into practice, providing options for optimal health, including cleansing, detoxifying, supplementation, lifestyle coaching, and homeopathic remedies.

Cindy is passionate about her journey to wellness and shares her experiences and knowledge with others as an inspiring speaker, educator, and practitioner.

Cindy was raised in Holland for the first part of her life, and then lived for 30 years in Ontario with her husband Glen, who is a Zen Shiatsu practitioner (Japanese Massage) and instructor of Yoga and Meditation. They share seven children between them. The couple presently reside and practice in the Bahamas.

INTRODUCTION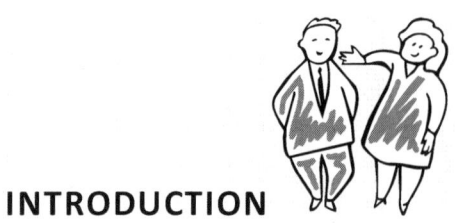

This book is designed to help you improve your hormone and breast health, therewith improving your overall health, which results in the prevention of disease, including breast cancer.

Health is the result of a combination of physical, mental, and spiritual aspects. My intent is to capture all these aspects in this guide.

Health is a result of educating yourself, to take responsibility for your body and mind, and to make educated lifestyle choices. You need to learn to look at prevention as a form of cure. Discovering that you are part of the decision-making process is *very* empowering.

This book is meant to *empower* you, to generate "informed consent", providing you with education and tools to take control of your life and health. This guide is developed as a tool. It can be used as a stand-alone tool for you to do the work by yourself, *or* you may choose to set up a series of coaching calls to help you become accountable for doing the "homework" at the end of this book and to hold you accountable for implementing the desired changes into your life.

I wish you much success on your health journey.

"For most people, cancer comes not from pre-programmed genes, but from conditions and exposures that are encountered throughout their life." Devra Lee Davis

TABLE OF CONTENTS

	Page
About the Author	i
Introduction	ii
Chapter 1: The Role of Informed Consent	**2**
What Does *Informed Consent* Mean?	2
What Should Be Involved in Informed Consent?	3
Chapter 2: The Role of Hormones in Breast Health	**6**
Hormone Health = Breast Health	6
What Are Hormones?	7
The Role of Estrogen and Progesterone in Breast Health	7
The Role of Bio-Identical Hormones in Breast Health	9
The Role of the Thyroid and Iodine in Breast Health	11
Chapter 3: The Role of Testing	**14**
Breast Self-Examination	15
Medical Breast Thermography	17
Mammograms, Ultrasounds, and MRIs	18
Hormone Testing	19
Iodine Testing	20
pH Alkalinity Testing	21
EMF Testing	23
Mercury and Heavy Metal Testing	23
Chapter 4: The Role of Diet and Nutrition	**23**
Prevention through Diet	23
Choose Organic Foods	24
Avoid Processed Foods	25
Avoid GMOs	25
Eliminate Hydrogenated Fats	27
Water and Water Filters	27
Decrease or Avoid Sugar	28
Sprouting and Juicing	28
Why Supplement, You Ask?	30
I-3-C, DIM and Calcium-D-Glucarate	32

Chapter 5: The Role of the Environment   34

    Environmental Links to Health and Wellness – Chart   35

Chapter 6: The Role of Detoxification   38

    Toxins   39
    The Lymphatic System   39
    How to Detoxify   42

Chapter 7: The Role of Emotions in Breast Health   44

    The Carcinogenic Personality   44
    Homeopathy to the Rescue   45
    Imagery and Visualization: Yoga, Meditation, and Self Image   47
    Is It Possible to Prevent Cancer?   48
    The Five "Wheels" of Total Health   49

Chapter 8: Your Complete 12-Step Action Plan   50

    How to have Happy Breasts   51
    Baby Steps – Your 12-Month Action Plan   52
    Personal Check List   60
    12-Month Calendar: Action List   61

Connect with Me Online   63

References and Resources   62

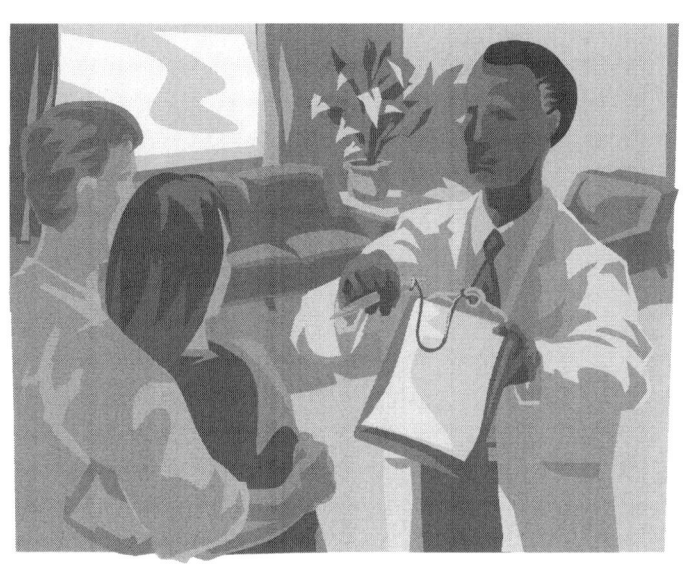

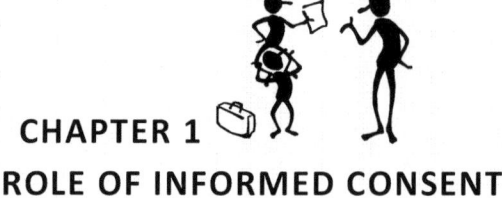

CHAPTER 1
THE ROLE OF INFORMED CONSENT

What Does *Informed Consent* Mean?

Informed consent is the method by which a <u>fully informed patient</u> can participate in choices about his or her health care. It comes from the legal and ethical right patients have to direct what happens to their body and from the ethical duty of the health care provider to involve patient in their own health care.

The <u>goal</u> of proper informed consent is to give patients the opportunity to be informed, active participants in their health care decisions. In international clinical research, it is standard practice that a patient signs a written Informed Consent form *after* he or she has been fully informed by the health care provider of the benefits and risks of the study or procedure they are considering. The same applies to any of your decisions when you are with your general practitioner (GP), specialist or at your hospital (or at your public schools, for that matter) when the use of medications, procedures, or operations is discussed. You should be aware that you have the <u>right</u> to be informed of the benefits, health risks, and side effects of a drug, procedure, or operation. Furthermore, you should be informed of reasonable alternative choices.

Don't be shy to ask your doctor for detailed information of the drug or procedure you are discussing. Take the information home, study and research it, and then go back for a second appointment with your decision. When discussing vaccinations and immunizations, ask your doctor for the Vaccine Information Statement (VIS). The Centers for Disease Control and Prevention (CDC) in North America produce Vaccine Information Statements to inform patients and their legal representatives of the benefits and risks of vaccines which are to be administered. The newest version must be used as it includes the most current and relevant information. If the patient or his/her parent or legal representative is unable to read or is limited by a physical disability, the VIS must be supplemented by visual aids or oral presentation. A health care provider, who follows proper informed consent processes and provides vaccine information, practices good management and good medical conduct.

What Should Be Involved in Informed Consent?

Informed consent involves:

- An explanation of the nature of the decision/procedure/medication
- Reasonable alternatives to the proposed intervention
- Related risks, benefits, and uncertainties to each alternative
- The physician assessing your understanding of this information prior to proceeding
- Your right to accept or turn down the intervention
- Voluntary (without coercion) consent

For surgery, anesthesia, and other invasive procedures, written informed consent is normally required. For other not-so-invasive procedures, verbal informed consent is needed and appropriate.

When medicine is recommended, the choice should be made by active and informed participation of the patient.

The requirements of informed consent are well known in moral principles and in law. For example, a chiropractor or medical doctor who is unable to obtain a patient's informed consent may be held accountable for battery (an unauthorized touching of the patient) or, more likely, for negligence (the negligent failure to make proper disclosure to the patient). Chiropractors and doctors have to deal with reprimands by their professional disciplinary bodies and are subject to penalties under provincial and state licensing legislation.

Informed consent is complete when:

- The patient has received information about a treatment, alternative courses of action, the material effects, the risks and side effects for each course of action, and the consequences of not having the treatment that a reasonable person in the same circumstances would require in order to make a decision
- The health care practitioner has responded to the patient's requests for other information about the treatment, alternative courses of action, material effects, risks and side effects, and consequences of not having the treatment.

This definition of informed consent should apply to both "medical" and "non-medical" procedures in a country, such as Canada, where 60% of the population use natural alternatives as part of their healthcare choices.

While individual governments press ahead with coercive vaccination policies, disrespecting medical ethics which protect the right of individuals to self determination around all medical procedures, the spirit and intent of medical law encourages the individual's right to independence and full participation in the decision-making process when considering treatment.

Repeatedly, patients find themselves intimidated or bullied into a decision, often against their own better judgment, and without the opportunity to satisfactorily consider all the risks involved.

According to The Ethics in Medicine from the University of Washington School of Medicine, the legal principles and ethics, which have come out of case law and Supreme Court decisions, consist of a body of knowledge that allows every individual the right to information on material risks and the fundamental right of persons to be free from unwanted physical interference. Medical care is unfair and a 'battery' unless the patient has given consent to it. It is a critical requirement to the demand of medical services.

Furthermore the University of Washington continues to state, the patient must understand the risks, no matter how statistically insignificant these may be. "When a patient reads, understands, and signs a written consent to treatment or surgery there is express consent. Express consent is established when a patient declares his willingness to submit to a medical treatment."

With regard to breast health, in order to have informed consent, women require information on the probabilities of different outcomes of various tests, medications (like Tamoxifen) and procedures (like mammography) in order to facilitate informed decisions.

Presently, women in North America do not go through the proper process of either written or verbal informed consent when it comes to mammograms or ultrasounds. Compulsory informed consent would allow women to make an informed decision, as is common practice for most other medical procedures. In the meantime, when you are at your doctor's office discussing breast health and screening options, ask your doctor to explain the risks, benefits, and alternatives. Then go home and think about this information and research it prior to giving consent.

MAINTAIN YOUR FREEDOM OF CHOICE:

BECOME INFORMED!

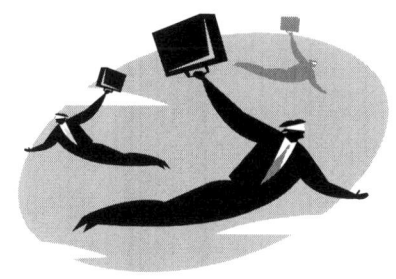

CHAPTER 2

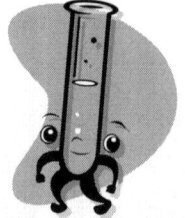

THE ROLE OF HORMONES IN BREAST HEALTH

Hormone Health = Breast Health

According to the National Cancer Institute, **90-95 % of breast cancers are lifestyle related.**

Hormone Health = Breast Health

Breast Health = Hormone Health

Hormonal Health is <u>key</u> in breast health <u>and</u> in overall health. Many women only find that out when they are diagnosed with breast cancer, at which point their tissue is tested for hormone levels. Eighty-Five percent (85%) of diagnosed breast cancers are *estrogen dominant*: **85%!** The reason your hormones are tested at the time of cancer is that the medical system now has a drug (like Tamoxifen) they can prescribe.

Why do they not test for hormones earlier in life, you ask? Well, preventatively speaking, they have no measures or drugs for the management of hormones. Now, however, more and more trained medical doctors specialize in the testing of hormones and use of bio-identical hormones.

Intuitively, many women realize how much hormones control their lives. From young teens, you experience the effects of hormones in sexual development, resulting in bodily changes. Most women understand hormones have something to do with teenage mood swings and menstrual symptoms. And you realize hormonal influences again going into pregnancy and menopause. Hormones control us from beginning to end, it seems. Therefore, breast health = hormone health, and *vice versa*.

When a woman's hormones are in proper balance, she feels great and has none of the symptoms she takes for granted during her menstrual cycles and in menopause.

What Are Hormones?

The word, *hormone*, comes from the Greek *Hormãn* = to set in motion, to stimulate.

Hormones are the chemical messengers of your body moving through the blood stream. Different hormones are produced by different glands.

Hormones are released when they receive the right triggers, which may be a chemical in the blood, another hormone, or xeno-hormone (a substance that mimics a hormone). Most hormones are proteins and steroids. Estrogen and progesterone are female sex hormones, which control a woman's monthly cycle.

The Role of Estrogen and Progesterone in Breast Health

Lorna R. Vanderhaeghe, MS refers to these hormones as your "sexy hormones". Other hormones, such as testosterone, dehydroepiandrosterone sulfate (DHEAS), and cortisol, are part of this group, however; estrogen and progesterone are the important hormones to focus on. I highly recommend her book, *Sexy Hormones*, if you feel inclined to learn all about hormones and the excellent products she recommends.

As mentioned before, 85% of breast cancers are diagnosed as <u>estrogen dominant</u>. What does this mean? In many cases, it means either too much estrogen (mostly estradiol) in your body or too little progesterone. Estrogen and progesterone work as a team and, therefore, the quotient percentage between them is very important to know and understand. Estrogen dominance puts a woman at greater risk for breast cancer, uterine fibroids, endometriosis, low sex drive, and ovarian cysts.

What is wrong with us, you ask, where so many women have too much estrogen in their body? Is it just your body malfunctioning, and if so, *why*? Many environmental factors influence and affect your hormones (hormone mimickers), such as cosmetics, plastics, water, dairy products, red meat, chicken, and pesticides. Synthetic estrogens found in birth control pills and fertility drugs contribute to estrogen overload.

Therefore, keeping your hormones balanced is not achieved just by taking a supplement, or by undergoing bio-identical hormone therapy. Balancing hormones should involve a multi-faceted approach, including lifestyle changes. The rest of this book is written to educate you on all these environmental and lifestyle factors so you can make educated choices going forward and, thereby, reducing your risk level of developing breast cancer.

Estrogen Facts

Here are some basic facts about estrogen that you should know:

- Estrogen is one of the many hormones in your body.
- 85% of breast cancer is estrogen dominant.
- All hormones are created (*or are supposed to be created*) in precise amounts in response to your body's need.
- Breast tissue contains a high amount of receptors for female hormones, especially estrogens.
- There are three main forms of estrogen: estradiol, estrone, and estriol.
- Even the weakest birth control pill contains *seven times* the amount of estrogen naturally occurring in your body.
- The ovaries produce most of your estrogens.
- Estrogen stimulates breast cells to multiply.
- "Traveling" estrogen can be recycled to be used again (you want to prevent this). This is more likely to occur in a diet high in saturated fat and meat.
- A diet high in fiber and plant lignans (flaxseed) reduces estrogen recycling.
- Vegetarians excrete two to three times <u>more</u> estrogen in their stools than non-vegetarians!
- Circulating estradiol and estrone levels are 50% higher in meat-eaters than in vegetarians.
- Balancing estrogen levels is essential in breast cancer prevention.
- Estrogen is derived from both internal and external environments.
- Estrogen dominance and progesterone deficiency are linked to cystic breasts, breast cancer, fibroids, cysts, endometriosis, and hypothyroidism.

Progesterone Facts

These progesterone facts help understand how this hormone works in the body:

- Progesterone is a *precursor* hormone, which means the body can use it to make other hormones, such as cortisol and dehydroepiandrosterone sulfate (DHEAS).
- Progesterone is the "feel-good" hormone during pregnancy, as it is high at this time.
- Progesterone, estrogen's "partner", protects from estrogen excess.
- Progesterone levels naturally decrease at menopause when the ovaries stop producing eggs.

The Estrogen – Progesterone Relationship

Let's look at what we know about the interaction of estrogen and progesterone:

- I repeat, estrogen's "partner" is progesterone, and it protects from estrogen excess.
- If estrogen levels are low, progesterone comes to the rescue by *converting* to estrogen.
- If estrogen levels are high, then you need more progesterone to keep the balance.
- Not only does stress cause progesterone to be unable to connect to its receptors, stress also creates more estrogen. You can see how stress can cause hormonal havoc.

How to Balance Estrogen and Progesterone

Use these means of balancing estrogen and progesterone:

- Check your hormone levels annually via saliva and blood samples.
- You can check your C-2 and C1-6 estrogen ratios via a urine test.
- Use ground flaxseed daily (grind the seeds yourself prior to each use).
- Use turmeric in your dishes.
- Supplement with indole-3-carbinol (I3C) or diindolymethane (DIM) to assist with estrogen balance.
- Supplement with calcium-D-glucarate and vitamin D.
- Consume a low-fat, high-fiber vegetarian diet, which includes wheat bran, psyllium, legumes, and flaxseed as part of a healthy breast diet.
- Supplement with wheat bran and psyllium, as these can help decrease circulating estrogen levels and prevent constipation.

The Role of Bio-Identical Hormones in Breast Health

Bio-Identical hormone (BIH) therapy is popular right now, and it seems like bio, or natural, hormones are an easy "fast fix". Personally, I feel that BIH therapy is a good choice <u>after</u> you have adopted all the other environmental and lifestyle changes in your life. If upon (re)testing, <u>after</u> you have made some drastic lifestyle changes, your hormones are still out of balance, perhaps the time has come to consider therapy with naturally derived hormones. Make sure you find a doctor specialized in bio-identical hormone treatment.

Hormone Replacement Therapy (HRT)

You've probably heard about synthetic hormones and bio-identical hormones. Let's explore the facts a bit about both.

- Hormone Replacement Therapy involves taking estrogen and progesterone orally.
- HRT is risky because these are *synthetic* molecules never before found in human bodies and therefore do not harmoniously interact with your cells.
- Synthetic HRT increases the risk of breast cancer. In 2002, a huge double-blind placebo study called "Women's Health Initiative" sponsored by the World Health Organization (WHO) was stopped early because it was proven during the study that HRT causes breast cancer.
- HRT has been used for menopausal and post-menopausal symptoms.

Natural Hormones

Read about why natural hormones are a better option:

- Natural, bio-identical hormones, on the other hand, are safe. They are hormones made from plant sources, including yam and soy, which are processed to mimic your own progesterone, estrogen, and testosterone. (Other hormones used can include DHEA and thyroid hormones).
- Bio-identical hormones such as estrogen, progesterone and testosterone, are precisely identical to those found in human bodies.

    CAUTION: Even safe, effective, natural hormone treatments should be monitored closely. Be sure you test regularly (preferably via blood *and* saliva, and monitor with thermography) and work with a Natural Health Care provider experienced and trained in hormones.

The Role of the Thyroid and Iodine in Breast Health

The thyroid gland releases three important hormones, known as T3, T4, and calcitonin. If the thyroid does not send out enough T3 and T4, you get symptoms of feeling cold and tired, dry skin, and weight gain (symptoms of *hypo*, or low, thyroid).

The job of the thyroid is to control the body's metabolic rate, which is the amount of energy expended in a given period and which affects how energetic you are.

Every organ in your body needs iodine, with the thyroid being the first to use any "incoming" iodine. The next biggest "customer" for iodine is your breast tissue. The problem is the low dietary intake of iodine in the North-American diet. Iodine prevents goiter (thyroid tumors), fibrocystic breast disease, and fatigue and depression due to thyroid insufficiency.

When thyroid function is low and the body can't work at its best, one consequence is that not enough estrogen is excreted and, therefore, a <u>surplus</u> of estrogen is the result, which can promote breast cancer.

Low Thyroid = High Estrogen = Keeps Thyroid Hormones Inactive

When testing your hormone levels with your doctor, ask him/her to check the FREE T-3 and FREE T-4 levels. In Canada and the USA, the *upper level of normal* for Thyroid Stimulating Hormone (TSH) is between 0.5 and 5.0 mU/l. According to Thyroid International 2008 (published by Merck in Germany), the definition of the reference range of TSH is of critical importance for the diagnosis. Cut-off levels of 0.3–0.4 mU/l for the lower limit of TSH and 4–5 mU/l for the upper one are conventionally used, however, a much lower upper limit of TSH was recently suggested, based on large population studies performed both in iodine-rich and iodine-deficient regions. Most naturopaths and natural health care practitioners agree that TSH levels above 2.0 are an early indication of *hypo*thyroid conditions.

Thyroid Issues are often a Pre-Cursor to Breast Conditions

According to Thyroid International, the same publication mentioned above, although the effects of iodine supply are regarded as small, experimental evidence in healthy subjects clearly demonstrates that short-term alterations in iodide availability may change TSH considerably, with a doubling of TSH levels three weeks after iodine treatment.

Furthermore, there is a direct relationship between your ovaries and the thyroid gland. The thyroid has and needs the greatest amount of iodine – the ovaries contain the 2nd largest concentration of iodine. Therefore if you are iodine deficient (which MOST North-American women are) it effects both your thyroid AND your ovaries.

In his book *Breast Cancer and Iodine*, Dr. David M. Derry, MD, PhD explores the role of iodine and the thyroid gland. This book is about cause, prevention, and treatment of breast cancer. According to his research, breast cancer has two phases. The first phase, from abnormal cells up to carcinoma *in situ*, reverses with iodine. The second phase, invasion, is controlled by connective tissue thyroid hormone.

The Japanese consume the highest amount of iodine in the world and have the lowest rate of breast cancer, prostate cancer, and thyroid cancer. Compared to the North-American diet, the Japanese diet has ten times more iodine in natural forms, such as seaweed and fish.

Iodine Facts

Take note of these iodine facts:

- Iodine is used to make thyroid hormone in the thyroid gland.
- Iodine triggers *apoptosis* (programmed cell death) in cells.
- Iodine detoxifies chemicals.
- Iodine is a great antiseptic to bacteria and viruses.
- A lack of iodine causes fibrocystic breast disease.

What You Can Do

Follow these steps to promote iodine efficiency:

- Use an infrared sauna program to remove toxins.
- Take daily amounts of selenium, zinc, vitamin B12, flaxseed oil, and tyrosine.
- Switch to using sea salt in your food preparations.
- If you are on Tamoxifen, use extra iodine and selenium.
- Have your iodine levels tested, and if low, supplement with kelp tablets, Lugol's iodine and/or sea vegetables. The foods richest in iodine are dulce and kelp.
- If you have mammograms, ask for the thyroid protection guard.

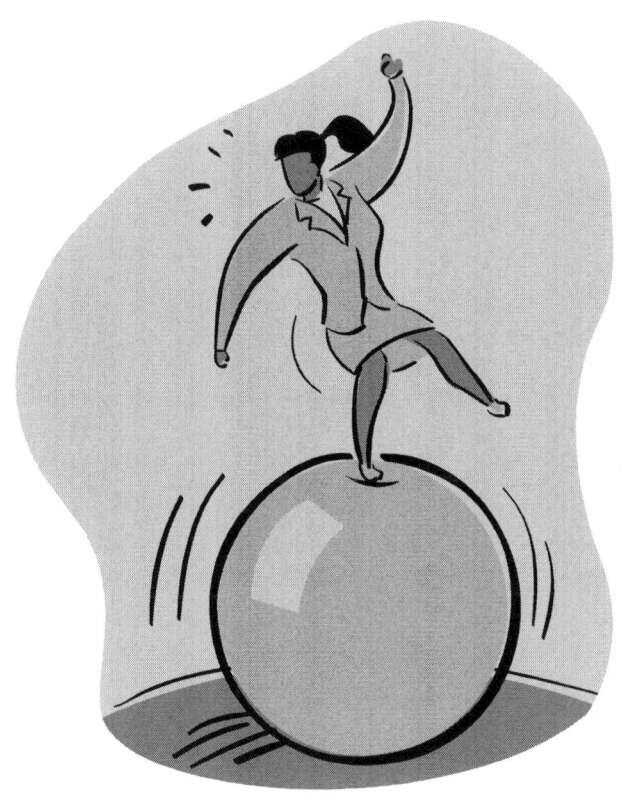

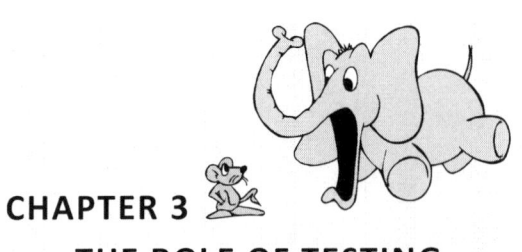

CHAPTER 3

THE ROLE OF TESTING

To test or not to test? Are we doing too many tests?

Does over-testing result in over-diagnosis and, therefore, over-treatment or unnecessary treatment?

As a classically trained homeopath, I ponder this question, as I understand the damage that fear and worry can do. For this reason, my opinion follows along the same lines as taking out different insurance policies: I choose the minimal necessary ones based on my signs, symptoms, and history, which may change from year to year.

As you are all individuals, you all react differently to what appears to be the same stimulus. As a breast thermography technician, meeting with each client to go over the reports, I have seen all kinds of responses. Some women just do it routinely and it does not affect them at all; others are physically ill prior to their appointment for fear of hearing "bad news". Thermography has a rating system from TH-1 (lowest risk) to TH-5 (highest risk). TH-2 is a normal low risk; however, I have encountered women who are devastated by this rating, which is considered a good rating. Subsequently, I may take a different approach to sharing information my clients or go slower or faster, depending on their particular sensitivity.

"And thereby some people are being treated for things which will never bother them, and yet they can be harmed by treatment," says Welch, author of *Overdiagnosed: Making People Sick in the Pursuit of Health*. Dr. Welch explains further in an interview in "Healthy Living Magazine" with the example that a simple blood test, the prostate-specific antigen test, or PSA test, was introduced 20 years ago. Now, 20 years later, about a million men are diagnosed with a cancer, which was never going to bother them.

I agree with Dr. Welch that, in the end, it comes down to finding the right balance for each individual. To be able to determine right balance for *you*, the reader, I will use this chapter to describe some of the tests, with their pros and cons, that I recommend to my patients. By no means do I suggest you do all of them, although that would be optimal.

Breast Self-Examination (BSE)

Statistics show that 70% of breast lumps are found by women themselves. Therefore, breast self-examination is a great, non-invasive diagnostic tool. It can be performed by your doctor, or you can implement a breast self-examination routine into your life by yourself, with your partner, or with a group of female friends. I suggest these various approaches, as I do understand that in many women breast examination creates a fear - the fear of finding a lump. See if you can find a way to implement regular breast self-examinations into your life in a non-fearful way.

There are many techniques for examining the breasts, and to use any is better than to use none at all. However, one method, which is very thorough, is the MammaCare Method (www.mammacare.com).

It is a carefully researched, systematic procedure, which brings sensitivity-trained finger pads in contact with every inch of the breast tissue. This exam can take several minutes. Do not be concerned; the exam is the most thorough you will have ever had.

In addition to covering the entire breast, one of the defining features of the MammaCare Method is the emphasis on multiple pressures to ensure contact with all depths of the breast tissue. This technique requires using deep pressure in some locations.

Women are told to do breast self-exams; however, if you do not know what to feel for or the best way to do your exam, the exam will not be very beneficial. MammaCare Breast Self-Exams enable a woman to exam her breasts with confidence. Training can raise the sensitivity of a woman's fingers to levels equal to or better than the sensitivity of the fingers of physicians, who have not been trained in the MammaCare Method.

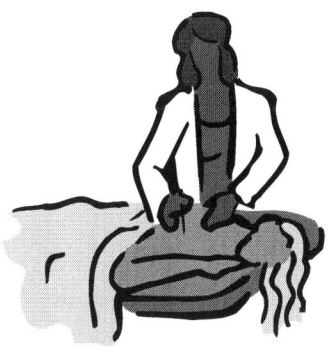

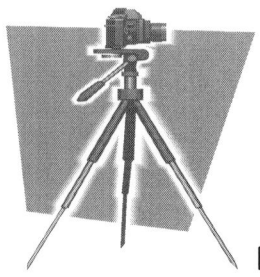

Medical Breast Thermography

Digital Infrared Scanning (breast thermography) is an FDA-approved assessment tool that is simple, painless, and uses no radiation.

When thermography is added to a multi-modal approach of breast exams, namely self-examination, examination by a doctor, and structural testing, 95% of early stage cancers can be detected.

What's more is that thermography is an early risk assessment of breast health. Breast thermography measures infrared radiation, in other words the heat or inflammation, which is constantly radiating, or emitting, away from the surface of the human skin. The infrared images show subtle temperature changes in the breast tissue. Blood supply, or vascularity, appears hyperthermic, or hot, and is depicted in thermographic images as red or white in color. Hypothermic, or cold, areas are depicted as darker, cooler colors in thermographic images. Normal breast tissue is displayed in varying shades.

Thermography is the most reliable form of early assessment. Though it is not often used in the medical field, it is becoming more readily available. Thermography has 90% sensitivity for both false positive and false negative readings. Thermography is painless and offers a view of the entire chest and underarm area. Nearly 50% of tumors are found in the upper chest or underarm areas - areas that mammograms don't cover.

Furthermore, thermography is an objective method to evaluate if therapies or lifestyle changes are actually working to reduce risk. For example, many women today use bio-identical hormones, which can be very beneficial. However, not all women react the same way to these treatments and thermography provides a way of measuring the results of treatment.

Thermography is a safe and effective exam for indicating:

- Inflammatory breast cancer
- Hormonal influence on the breast tissue
- Fibrocystic activity or conditions
- Thyroid-related conditions
- Monitoring of hormone replacement therapy
- Undetected dental inflammation and TMJ issues
- Vascular disease

The chart below describes the growth rate of cancer cells, indicating the early stage that thermography picks up signs of risk compared to when a mammogram detects a lump:

Active Cancer Cells Double in Number Every 90 Days

90 days	2 cells	
1 year	16 cells	
2 years	256 cells	→ Thermography detects changes
3 years	4,896 cells	
4 years	65,536 cells	
5 years	1,08,576 cells	→ Changes still undetectable by a mammogram
6 years	16,777,216 cells	
7 years	268,435,456 cells	(Size has doubled 32 times)*
8 years	4,294,967,296 cells	

*Normally detectable by mammogram at this stage

40 Doublings (approx. 10 years) is considered lethal

Source: Buchanan, J.B. et al., "Tumor Growth, doubling time, and inability of the radiologist to diagnose certain cancers."

Mammograms, Ultrasounds, and MRIs

The real problem is that most breast cancers develop for up to 8-10 years *before* a palpable lump can be found or detected by mammography or other structural tests. This fact is not well understood by most women and, therefore, they are often mislead to believe that mammography, ultrasounds, and MRIs are the best thing they can do to monitor their breast health. In other words, a woman may actually have breast cancer, but it goes undetected because her lesion is too small to be seen by a mammogram or because her breasts are too dense to even provide a reliable mammogram.

Both mammography and ultrasound are structural, or anatomical, tests, while thermography is a functional, or physiological, test.

Please understand the difference between a *screening* mammogram and a *diagnostic* mammogram. Screening mammograms are those performed on healthy women routinely on an annual or bi-annual basis. Diagnostic mammograms are those ordered specifically when there are particular concerns and symptoms.

Mammogram Facts

Take note of these little mammogram facts and go see the Fact Sheet on Mammograms by the National Cancer Institute

- Mammograms expose your body to radiation, which can be 1,000 times greater than that from a regular chest X-ray, and which poses risks of cancer.
- Mammography compresses the breasts tightly, and often painfully, which can lead to a lethal spread of malignant cells.
- Cancers are often missed in pre-menopausal women, who have dense breasts, and postmenopausal women on estrogen replacement therapy.
- False diagnoses are common, and women may be unnecessarily caused to worry and experience anxiety.

"OUR CURRENT ESTIMATE IS THAT ABOUT 75% OF THE CURRENT ANNUAL INCIDENCE OF BREAST CANCER IN NORTH AMERICA IS BEING CAUSED BY EARLIER IONIZING RADIATION, PRIMARILY FROM MEDICAL SOURCES."

John W. Goffman, MD, PhD; Committee for Nuclear Responsibility in Preventing Breast Cancer: The Story of a Major, Proven, Preventable Cause of This Disease

Hormone Testing

As you have by now learned, balancing your hormones is a large part of your breast health. Therefore, let's discuss which hormones should be tested and the pros and cons of the methods most commonly used.

Hormone testing is a combination of your menstrual history, your signs and symptoms, and blood and/or saliva testing.

Annual testing of the following hormones is recommended:

- Estrogen (Estradiol, Estrone, Estriol)
- Progesterone
- DHEAS
- Melatonin
- IGF-1
- Cortisol
- Testosterone
- Vitamin D
- For Thyroid: TSH, Free T3, Free T4 and thyroid antibodies

Blood Hormone Tests

Blood levels of estradiol FSH, LH, progesterone, testosterone, and DHEAS can give an indication of hormonal imbalance. Blood hormone tests are limited because they measure the hormones bound to blood proteins, which are your inactive hormones. Estriol can be measured with a 24-hour urine test or with saliva.

It is best to first have your blood hormone levels checked by your doctor and then arrange a saliva hormone test for a more accurate evaluation of your hormone levels. Saliva tests provide the bio-available levels of hormones in your system.

Saliva Hormone Tests

Hormones have been measured in saliva for over 30 years, and research continues to accumulate attesting to saliva testing's reliability and clinical relevance. Despite a wealth of supporting evidence, many are still critical of saliva hormone testing. These criticisms have arisen largely from misuse of the test results - specifically, by reading too much into what the numbers mean. Saliva hormone testing is very useful for finding underlying hormone excesses and deficiencies, but needs to be interpreted with care when hormones are being supplemented.

Basal Body Temperature Tests

Basal body temperature tests are used for assessing thyroid function. You can monitor your basal temperature at home as a simple, inexpensive way to evaluate your thyroid function.

Plan to measure your temperature as soon as you wake up in the morning <u>before</u> rising. You have to shake down the basal thermometer the night before and leave it at your bedside.

Procedure

1. Take your temperature in your armpit for *10 minutes* first thing in the morning <u>before</u> you get up. (Normal temperature is 36.6 C – 36.8 C.).
2. Record daily temperatures on a chart for 14 days.
3. Mark the first day and the last day of your menstrual period on the chart with an X. Your temperature will usually be higher the last two weeks of your cycle.
4. If your temperature is consistently <u>lower than 36.6 C</u>, you may have an underactive thyroid, underactive adrenals, low progesterone, low iron levels or a combination of any of these.

Iodine Testing

Let's take a closer look at the various tests available.

Iodine Loading Tests

This test's normal values are based on seeing if the person is deficient in iodine or iodide. A sample of urine is taken as an early morning void to measure the level of iodine before loading. This is known as a SPOT test and it establishes the baseline value for the person. Next the patient is given 50 mg of iodine as a loading dose. A 24-hour urine collection for the amount of iodine or iodide excreted is taken after this load dose. This test compares the urinary iodine values to the normal creatinine value which is excreted by the kidney in urine. Creatinine is a byproduct of muscle metabolism and is an indicator of kidney function.

Iodine Test in Dried Urine

In this test, Iodine is collected twice during the day (first morning and last night void) on filter strips either by dipping the strip in urine collected in a cup, or by urinating directly on the strip. The urine-saturated filter strips are allowed to dry overnight and then sent to the laboratory for iodine and creatinine testing. Iodine is expressed as the average of morning and night levels per liter urine and mg creatinine.

Iodine Patch Tests

This method is the simplest and least expensive. The only material you need is Tincture of Iodine, the original colored solution, not the clear one. Paint a swatch of the iodine over your stomach, approximately three inches in diameter, and then observe how long it takes the color to fade from your skin. The faster the color fades, the greater the chance of iodine deficiency. It's a sign of severe iodine deficiency if the color fades in less than four hours. If the color remains after 24 hours, then it's likely you are iodine sufficient.

However, according to Dr. David Derry, MD and author of the book, *Breast Cancer and Iodine*, the iodine patch test is not a is not an indicator of anything: *"The iodine disappearance rate is unrelated to thyroid disease or even iodine content of the body. (1-2) Meticulous research by Nyiri and Jannitti in 1932 showed clearly when iodine is applied to the skin in almost any form, 50% evaporates into the air within 2 hours and between 75 and 80 percent evaporates into the air within 24 hours. (1) A total of 88 percent evaporates within 3 days and it is at this point that the evaporation stops. The remaining 12 percent that is absorbed into the skin has several fates. Only 1-4% of the total iodine applied to the skin is absorbed into the blood stream within the first few hours. The rest of the iodine within the skin (8-11%) is slowly released from the skin into the blood stream."*

pH Alkalinity Testing

Your body maintains a very important pH balance, which needs to be upheld the best we can. However, both the water supply and food supply today are highly acidic. Cancer cells thrive in an acidic environment; therefore, striving for a pH of around 7.0 is your goal here.

Adjusting Your Acid and Alkaline Balance

This information can help you undertake steps to balance your alkalinity:

- The body makes an effort to maintain a 7.4 pH (potential of hydrogen).
- Cancer does not thrive in an alkaline environment (tumor cells die at a pH of 8).
- Alkaline minerals, which neutralize acids, are sodium, potassium, calcium, and magnesium.
- All animal foods are acid forming, as are most grains.
- Coffee, alcohol, sugar, drugs, refined foods, and meat all promote acidity.
- Fruits and vegetables are alkaline forming.

pH Tests

The two ways to monitor your pH are testing your saliva and testing your urine. You will need pH-testing strips, which are available from most pharmacies, from Amazon.com, or from your naturopathic doctor. Normal saliva pH levels should range from 6.4 to 7.2. Optimum levels should range from 6.6 to 6.8.

Saliva Test Procedure

1. Test your saliva first thing in the morning when you get out of bed.
2. Tear off a 1.5" strip of test paper.
3. Insert one end of the strip under your tongue, and wet it well.
4. Withdraw the strip, immediately compare its color to the color chart provided, and record the value. Your pH should be 6.8.
5. Check your saliva pH once more five minutes after breakfast. Ideally it should be 8.5 at that point.

Urine Test Procedure

Check the pH of your first and second urination of the day. Normal urine pH levels should range from 5.0 to 7.0. Optimum levels should range from 6.0 to 6.4.

1. Tear off a 1.5" of strip of test paper.
2. Dip one end of the strip in urine.
3. Draw the strip over the edge of the container as you withdraw it to remove excess urine.
4. Immediately compare the strip's color to the color chart provided, and record the value. The first test should be more acidic. The second test should be 6.8.

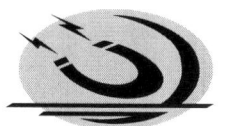

EMF Testing

Electro Magnetic Field (EMF) is a broad term which includes electric fields generated by charged particles, magnetic fields generated by charged particles in motion, and radiated fields, such as TV, radio, and microwaves, cell phones, computers, alarm clocks, etc.

DID YOU KNOW THAT THE WORLD HEALTH ORGANISATION CLASSIFIED THE RADIATION USED IN WI-FI AS POSSIBLY CARCINOGENIC?

Consider having an EMF Home Inspection and Consultation and reduce your family's in-home EMF exposure by up to 95% with an EMF survey, site inspection, and report. Contact www.EMFSolutions.ca in Canada.

There are filters, such as Graham-Stetzer filters, which can be installed to minimize EMF radiation.

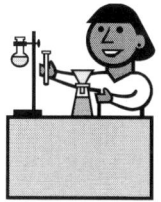

Mercury and Heavy Metal Testing

Two tests for mercury and heavy metals in the body analyze the urine or the hair.

Urine Toxic Metals Test

Analysis of the levels of toxic metals in urine after the administration of a metal detoxification agent is an objective way to evaluate the accumulation of toxic metals. Acute metal poisoning is rare. More common, however, is a chronic, low-level exposure to toxic metals, which can result in significant retention in the body, which can be associated with a vast array of adverse health effects and not chronic disease.

Hair Toxic Elements Test (Hair Analysis)

Extensive research has established that element levels in scalp hair are related to human systemic levels. The strength of this relationship varies for specific elements, and many researchers consider hair as the tissue of choice for toxic and several nutrient elements.

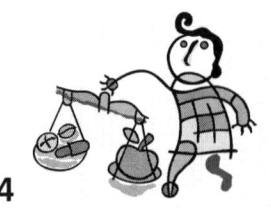

CHAPTER 4

THE ROLE OF DIET AND NUTRITION

It seems far-fetched to many people that what you eat can affect your breast and hormone health. However, remember we said earlier that your breast health is very much dependent on your hormonal balance and that 85% of breast cancers are estrogen dominant? If you eat the regular (non-organic) food supply, you are basically feeding yourselves a nutrient-poor and pesticide-rich diet. Many of these pesticides, herbicides, and chemicals affect your hormonal balance and, therefore. your breast health.

You **definitely** ARE what you EAT (and drink).

Prevention through Diet

Your goal is to consume "clean" (organic) food and water in its most natural form (raw). Cooked food loses most of the nutrients needed when cooked over 105 degrees Celsius. You should strive to eat and drink 80% alkaline and 20% acidic foods and water, as you now know that cancer can't thrive in an alkaline environment.

In summary, your goal is to:

- Consume organic food
- Eat 80% of your food uncooked, or raw
- Avoid processed foods
- Avoid Genetically Modified Organisms (GMOs)
- Eliminate hydrogenated fats
- Decrease, or avoid, sugar
- Strive for a balance of 80% alkaline and 20% acidic foods

DID YOU KNOW? ORGANIC VEGETABLE AND FRUIT LABEL CODES START WITH A 9.

Choose Organic Foods

Certain herbicides and pesticides on produce, as well as hormones found in conventional meats, are implicated in breast cancer. Eat more raw and organic vegetables from the Brassica family: broccoli, cabbage, Brussels sprouts, kale, and collard greens. The plant compounds they contain make estrogen less dangerous to breast tissue. Choose to eat them raw, when possible, to preserve nutrients.

NOTE: In their phenomenal bestseller, *Foods That Fight Cancer: Preventing Cancer Through Diet,* written by Montreal biochemist, Richard Beliveau, with fellow scientist Denis Gingras, the authors refer to fruits and vegetables as a preventative non-toxic version of chemotherapy.

Avoid Processed Foods

Refined carbohydrates, processed meats (hot dogs, sausage, etc) are proven to increase cancer risk. Processed foods include anything in a box or package that doesn't look like it just came from a farm!

Processed foods contain saturated fats, trans fats, refined carbohydrates, and preservatives, which actually increase inflammation throughout your body. Many processed foods contain white flour - be sure to avoid white flour, white rice and white breads. Eating processed foods has been proven to raise cancer risk in women, such as breast cancer, pancreatic, urinary tract and uterine cancer.

Replace luncheon meats with home-roasted organic meats. Roast a local, organic chicken once a week, and have chicken salad, roasted chicken sandwiches, and chicken soup for lunch instead of processed luncheon meats. A few times a week, choose to eat a vegetarian salad or sandwich.

Avoid GMOs

Genetically modified organisms (GMOs) use a laboratory process of artificially inserting genes into the DNA of food crops. These genes are obtained from bacteria, viruses, insects, animals, or even humans.

At present, in North America, no label is required to identify a GMO product; however, some products may have "non-GMO" labels.

GMO food is labeled or banned in: Europe, Japan, China, India, Russia, Brazil, Australia, Peru, and many other countries, however, not yet in North America.

Most genetically modified ingredients are products made from the *Big Four*:

- **Corn:** corn flour, meal, oil, starch, gluten and syrup, fructose, dextrose, glucose, and modified cornstarch
- **Soybeans:** soy flour, lecithin, protein, isolate, and vegetable oil
- **Canola:** oil (aka rapeseed oil)
- **Cottonseed**

GMO Agriculture Is the Opposite of Sustainable

Chances are you are already eating genetically engineered ingredients. Look at the labels on any of your packaged foods.

- Very few fresh fruits and vegetables are GMOs (only papaya from Hawaii).
- No genetically modified fish, fowl or livestock is yet approved for human consumption; however, many animals are raised on genetically modified feed, such as grains. Look for wild fish, rather than farmed.
- Some eggs are GMOs. Stick with organic eggs.
- Milk or soy protein is the basis for most infant formulas.
- Cereals and breakfast bars are very likely to include genetically modified ingredients, including soy and corn products.
- Many packaged breads and bakery items contain genetically modified ingredients, such as corn syrup.
- Many frozen foods are highly processed. Look for organic or non-GMO labels.
- Many soups and sauces are highly processed.
- Choose pure olive and coconut oils. Choose preserves, jams and jellies made with cane sugar, not corn syrup.
- Look for snacks made from wheat, rice, or oats and ones that use sunflower or safflower oils.
- Most juices, except papaya, are made from GMO-free fruit; however; the use of high fructose corn syrup in fruit juices is cause for concern. Many sodas and fruit beverages are mostly comprised of water and corn syrup. Look for 100% juice blends.

Dr. David Suzuki, noted Canadian environmentalist, and hundreds of other scientists have warned about the dangers of GMOs and their effects, not only on human health, but also on biodiversity. Our bees are dying, and as Einstein has stated, "If the bee disappeared off the surface of the globe, then man would only have four years of life left. No more bees, no more pollination, no more plants, no more animals, no more man."

Eliminate Hydrogenated Fats

Hydrogenated fats increase the risk of breast cancer. In fact, all oils that are altered through processing are toxic. On the other hand, oils with omega-3 fatty acids protect us from breast cancer. Why? Omega-3 fats weaken the effect of estrogen on breast cells and balance the tumor-promoting effects of Omega-6.

Consider these tips when shopping for oils:

- Choose organic butter instead of margarine.
- Use olive oil, coconut oil, or flax oil instead of refined oils.
- When buying oil, look for cold pressed.
- Saturated fats in meat, butter, animal products, and peanut oil increase breast cancer risk, so limit their consumption.
- Persons with cancer may need to take higher amounts of good quality, fresh flaxseed, and pure fish oil, and avoid Omega-6 oils until the cancer retreats.

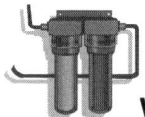

Water and Water Filters

The human body consists of 75% water. **Think about it!** The body has its own water regulating system, and without the proper quality and quantity of water, you create stressed organs. Water really is your foundation. Water in your bodies distributes the nutrients and excretes the toxins, some very important functions. Most water "out there" has low pH. In fact, the Japanese call it Dead Water. The pH of water should preferably be above 7.5, like the pH found in Kangen Water. Did you know that bottled water, such as Dasani, bottled by the Coca-Cola Company, has a pH of 4.5?

An Associated Press investigation shows that a vast array of pharmaceuticals - including antibiotics, anticonvulsants, mood stabilizers, and sex hormones - are found in the drinking water supplies of at least 41 million North Americans. In Canada, a national research institute found nine different drugs in water samples taken from 20 Ontario drinking water treatment plants.

Many health problems are related to chronic dehydration. Therefore, make an extra effort and start with a simple thing by drinking plenty of clean water. Even headaches and constipation can be due to a lack of water. Use a quality water filter, as the chlorine and fluoride in tap water have possible links to cancer. Drink healthy, alkaline drinking water with a high pH rating. Your drinking water should be rich in minerals, purged of impurities, and free of contamination.

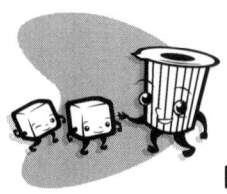

Decrease or Avoid Sugar

Author, Dr. Raymond Francis, states, "Here's the problem: The human body was simply not designed to handle refined sugars. They bring about a deadly combination of malnutrition and toxicity."

Read these sugar facts to understand why you should reduce your sugar intake:

- Sugar depresses the immune system.
- The rise of chronic disease in modern societies has paralleled the rise in sugar consumption.
- Sugar-induced hormone imbalances tax and weaken the immune system to the point where it can no longer defend the body.
- The refining process of sugar, making it white, removes 80- 90% of the chromium, manganese, cobalt, copper and zinc found in natural sugar.

What about sugar alternatives? Avoid aspartame! Aspartame is the technical name for Nutrasweet, Equal and Spoonfool and injures nervous tissue on a cellular level. Avoid Splenda (Sucralose) too while you are at it and choose a natural alternative. Sugar alternatives, like stevia and xylitol, are good substitutes

A diet high in fiber has been shown to remove toxic and carcinogenic substances from your bodies.

Fiber binds to hormones, like estrogen, and removes them from the body. Without fiber, the estrogen may be reabsorbed and excess estrogen is known to cause disease.

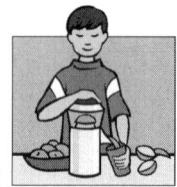

Sprouting and Juicing

Keeping your menu to liquids and green juices in the morning is an excellent way to aid your body's natural repair cycles.

Since your body is usually far too acidic, this is a good way to help flush out all the bad things and replace them with the good ones you need.

Juicing is the easiest and healthiest way to get in your daily intake of fruit and veggies in just one simple glass.

Juice Ingredients

You don't need to measure...just throw everything in the juicer!

- Celery-cucumber-carrots-apple
- Celery-cucumber-kale-apples
- Celery-kale-apple

Start small and simple and, eventually, you'll venture into all kinds of veggies and fruits!

Adding a sea-vegetable or green to your power juice is a great idea such as spirulina or chlorella.

Did you know?

- Fresh pineapple juice reduces arthritis swelling and inflammation.
- A smoothie of papaya, peppermint, and fennel relieves indigestion faster than the top-selling antacid.
- Eating lots of fresh fruit can reduce the incidence of psoriasis.

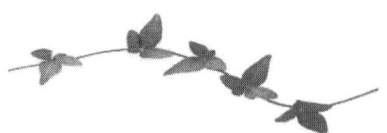

The Benefits of Sprouting

Sprouts are one of the most alkalizing, nutritious, and easily accessible foods known to man. Rich in vitamins, minerals, proteins, and enzymes, sprouts can be grown easily in 4-6 days, require no effort, and have very little cost.

The main benefit of sprouting is that it takes a seed or nut in the dormant state and brings it to life. During the sprouting process, new and higher quality proteins and other nutrients are produced.

Tests have shown that nutrients in seeds and nuts are anywhere from 50% to 400% greater after sprouting or soaking.

Step-by-Step Manual Sprouting

1. Place seeds in a sieve and wash thoroughly.
2. Soak the seeds overnight or for approximately 12 hours, and then rinse thoroughly.
3. Place the seeds in a germinator, and ensure they are evenly spread out and not too cramped together.
4. Place the germinator in a well-lit spot away from direct sunlight, and keep at room temperature.
5. Water twice daily.
6. After 4-6 days, your sprouts are ready to harvest – rinse thoroughly, and keep refrigerated. Consume within 5 days.

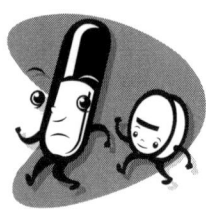

WHY SUPPLEMENT, YOU ASK?

Your body is unable to make most vitamins. Therefore, you must get them from what you eat or ingest. Many things in your environment deplete nutrients from your body. Physical and emotional stress, pollution, inadequate sleep, smoking, over-the-counter and prescription drugs, caffeine, and alcohol are the major environmental contributors that deplete our nutrients. Much of the food on the market lacks adequate nutritional value. Even the soil you grow your foods in is nutrient-poor.

Ever wonder what they mean by anti-oxidants and free radicals? Let me explain:

Anti-Oxidant: An anti-oxidant is any vitamin, mineral, or other nutrient that works against the cell-damaging process called oxidation (comparable to rust).

Oxidation: Oxidation is the gain of oxygen. Redox, or reduction-oxidation, is the loss of oxygen.

Free Radicals: Free radicals are atoms or groups of atoms that can cause damage to cells, impair the immune system and lead to infections and various diseases Free radicals are found in harmful substances such as cigarettes, some toxic chemicals, radiation, fried and processed foods and other pollutants.

The Benefits of Vitamins

Of course we know vitamins are good for us. Read on to learn their benefits:

- Without vitamins, enzymes can't work.
- Vitamin A helps to improve tissue tolerance for women undergoing chemotherapy.
- Beta-carotene has been shown to reduce the risk of pre-menopausal breast cancer by up to 90%.
- An excess of estrogen can deplete B vitamins.
- Vitamin B3 (niacin) is crucial in preventing the start of cancer and in reversing cancer.
- Vitamin B6 helps with good and harmful estrogen production.
- Vitamin IP6 (part of the B vitamins) acts to prevent cancer as it regulates cell division.
- Vitamin C can help reduce the risk of breast cancer.
- Vitamin E has been shown to decrease risk of breast cancer.

Minerals – How Important Are They?

Minerals are essential for your health, forming your bones, present in your muscles, blood, and nerve cells. The body utilizes over 80 minerals for maximum function. Even if you eat the healthiest foods, you are not getting all the minerals you need. Evidence of mineral malnutrition presents various minor and serious health conditions, such as energy loss, premature aging, diminished senses, and degenerative diseases like osteoporosis, heart disease and cancer. In many cases, these can be prevented with proper mineral supplementation.

Some **major minerals** our bodies need are: sodium, potassium, calcium, phosphorus, magnesium, manganese, sulfur, cobalt and chlorine. Our bodies also need **trace minerals** to function optimally. Examples of trace minerals are: iron, zinc, copper, selenium, iodine, fluorine, boron, and chromium. Many vitamins and minerals interact, working alongside each other in groups. For example, healthy bones require a good balance of vitamin D, calcium, phosphorus, magnesium, zinc, fluoride, chloride, manganese, copper, and sulfur.

Many of these elements can enhance or impair another vitamin's or mineral's absorption and functioning, For example, an excessive amount of iron can cause a deficiency in zinc.

Calcium and magnesium work together. Low calcium and vitamin D with a high fat diet causes a doubling of breast cancer incidences. Sugar, caffeine, salt, soft drinks, and excess protein deplete calcium.

Potassium keeps the body more alkaline, which is important because cancer prefers an acid body. Potassium stimulates the kidneys to eliminate waste.

Selenium deficiency has been linked with higher cancer incidence. Selenium reduces tumor size and stimulates your natural killer cells to directly target cancer cells, which we all have in our bodies. Furthermore, selenium is important for the conversion of T3 to T4 for your thyroid.

I-3-C, DIM and Calcium-D-Glucarate

Indole-3-Carbinol (I-3-C) is an anti-cancer phytonutrient found in cruciferous vegetables like broccoli, brussel sprouts, cauliflower, bok choi, kale, and cabbage. I-3-C promotes the formation of "good" estrogen. It inhibits human breast cancer cells from growing by as much as 90 %!

Research has shown I-3-C to be effective in breaking down cancer-causing estrogens in the liver into non-toxic forms, versus blocking them as Tamoxifen and other cancer drugs do. A research study appearing In "Cancer Watch" (2006, issue 4) showed that women on Tamoxifen needed less of the drug if they supplemented with indole-3-carbinol, delivering the same benefits whilst reducing side effects.

For those taking Tamoxifen, be aware of the side effects, which include hot flashes, nausea and vomiting, bone pain, diarrhea, irregular menstruation, skin rashes, tumor pain, vaginal bleeding, and vaginal discharge.

Diindolymethane (DIM) is a derivative of I-3-C. DIM forms naturally in the stomach when I3C is ingested.

Calcium-D-Glucarate is another powerful detoxifier of excess estrogens in the liver. Calcium-D-Glucarate is a botanical extract found in products, such as apples, oranges, grapefruit, Brussels sprouts, and broccoli. Scientists have noted that this supplement appears to protect against cancers and other degenerative diseases in a manner different than the traditional antioxidants. It has been shown to include regulation of estrogen metabolism and as a lipid-lowering agent.

Check to see if *your* supplementation includes these beneficial nutrients.

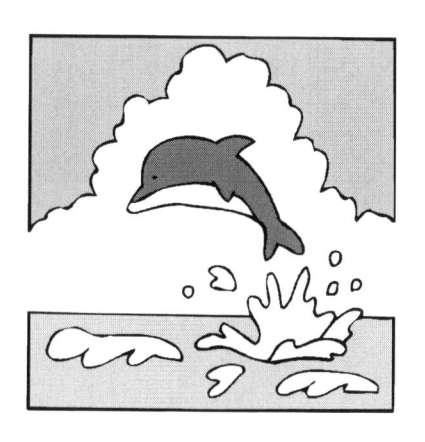

Studies show that ocean water contains approximately 90 elements, in the correct proportions, needed BY THE HUMAN BODY.

CHAPTER 5
THE ROLE OF THE ENVIRONMENT

Environment: the aggregate of surrounding things, conditions, or influences; surroundings; milieu

Ecology: the air, water, minerals, organisms, and all other external factors surrounding and affecting a given organism at any time - the social and cultural forces that shape the life of a person or a population

Do you think your environment affects your hormones? There is a lot more media and information now about the effects of chemicals in your food, water, and household goods. Specifically, estrogen-mimicking chemicals are of concern to us in dealing with breast health. Indeed, the chemical environment affects your cells and your hormones.

Some Resources:
- www.cosmeticsdatabase.com for cosmetics
- www.lesstoxicguide.ca guide for less toxic household products
- www.thegreenguide.com for everyday living
- www.organiclawncaretips.com for pesticides and fertilizers
- www.DirtyElectricity.ca for EMF information and inspections
- Book: *Healing the Planet, One Patient at a Time* by Jozef J. Krop, MD, FAAEM A primer in Environmental Medicine
- Book: *Make Home Safe Home* by Debra Lynn Dadd

Natural Household Alternatives

Use these healthier, alternative, cleaning products in your home:
- White Vinegar - disinfects and deodorizes
- Lemon Juice - cuts grease & polishes metal
- Washing Soda - general cleaning and deodorizing
- Borax - kills mold
- Olive oil - mix with vinegar for furniture polish
- Alka-Seltzer – cleans toilets
- Club Soda and Salt: removes carpet stains. You can also try a three-to-one mixture of vinegar and water and pouring the mixture onto the stains
- Corn Gluten Meal or "Turf Maize": kills weeds. You can also pour boiling water between patio stones to kill weeds.

Environmental Links to Health and Wellness

Each year, an additional 1,000 new chemicals are developed and introduced into your environment.

The following table lists common environmental elements that affect your health:

Environmental Element	Health Effects
Electro Magnetic Fields (EMFs)	Electricity and EMFs are linked to an increase in breast cancer. EMFs are present in wiring, phones, computers, TVs, fridges, hairdryers, clocks, and ovens. Exposure disturbs the growth pattern of cells and creates DNA damage, and results in deficiency in melatonin, which results in increase of breast cancer. Frequent use of cell phones has been linked to headaches, fatigue, dizziness, and brain tumors.
Household Cleaning Products	Many household products contain formaldehyde, chlorides, reproductive toxins, or hormone disruptors, which can cause liver, kidney, and brain damage, allergies and asthma. Hormone disrupting parabens may be used as preservatives.
Personal Care Products (For Men, Too)	Many personal care products you use daily can be hazardous to your health. These include toothpaste, cosmetics, hand creams, fragrances, shampoos, soaps, deodorants, and hair dyes. Cosmetics and toiletries sometimes contain a potentially dangerous mix of carcinogens, mutagens, and reproductive toxins, which can alter the function of hormones.
Pesticides and Chemical Fertilizers	Most gardeners use chemicals to fertilize plants and to fight pests and diseases. This destroys helpful soil organisms and can damage a plant's natural ability to fend off pests and diseases. Herbicides and pesticides kill bees and other pollinators.

Environmental Element	Health Effects
Plastics: Plexiglas, latex, nylon, polyester, polyurethane, Polyvinyl chloride (PVC), Polyvinylpyrrolidone (PVP) used in hairsprays, teflon, and styrofoam	PVC is responsible for the greatest production and use of chlorine. Used in cars, toys, food containers, credit cards, raincoats, wallpaper, furniture, building supplies, water pipes, windows, flooring. Dioxins and phthalates are often added to PVC and are hormone-disrupting chemicals Chemicals like phthalates and bisphenol-A (BPA) are added to plastic keep it soft and flexible, used in toys, water bottles, soup cans etc. These plasticizers contaminate food. Release of toxins from plastic wrap and plastic containers is made worse when the material is heated, as in a microwave, or when a plastic water bottle is left in a hot car.
Radiation	<ul><li>Radiation depletes white blood count and depresses immunity. As a result, free radicals form, and these deform your red blood cells.</li><li>Airplanes give off radiation. A flight of 6 hours exposes you to 5 millirads of radiation.</li><li>Chest X-rays expose you to 16 millirads of radiation each time.</li><li>Mammograms expose you to 1,000 times more rads than a normal chest X-ray!</li><li>Note: This type of radiation is cumulative, which means it adds up each time you are exposed.</li></ul>
Your Drinking Water	Fluoride in your water causes low thyroid conditions because it inhibits the thyroid hormone. Fluoride is found in fluoridated toothpaste, dental treatments, mouth rinses, baby vitamins, and fruit juices, where water is added from fluoridated sources. Fluoride is an acute toxin with a rating slightly higher than lead. Fluoride is banned in Sweden, Norway, Denmark, Germany, Italy, Belgium, Austria, France, and Holland. Chlorine in your drinking water causes cancer. Essentially, it's bleach.

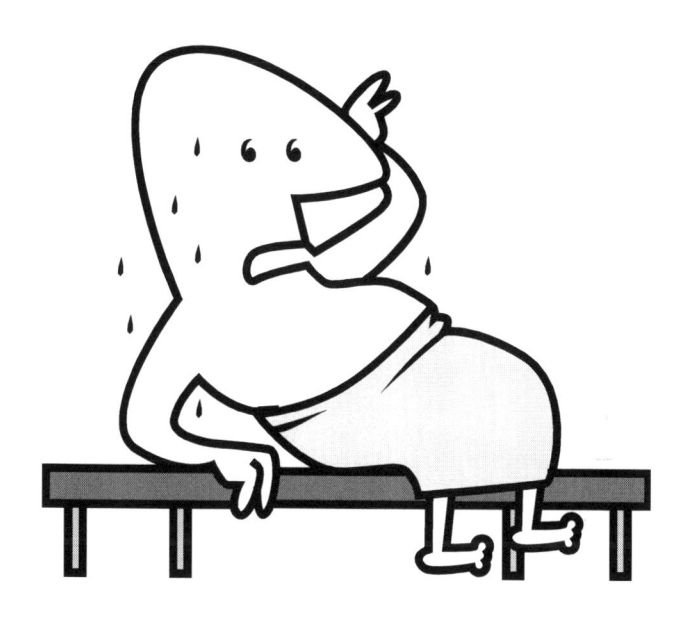

CHAPTER 6
THE ROLE OF DETOXIFICATION

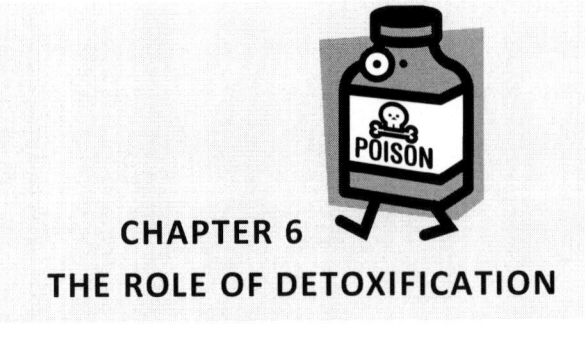

Reducing toxic overload is <u>key</u> to eliminating cancer.

Cancer is caused by environmental toxins. (Refer to the previous chapter for details.) Since the Second World War, over 100,000 chemicals have been introduced into your environment and your bodies. Your immune and defense systems are simply overwhelmed by the amount of toxins. There are a variety of toxicities, which can build up.

We'll outline two of them here:

- **Cellular toxicity** is created by the acidity in your bodies.
- **Heavy metal toxicity** comes from the metals you are exposed to. For example, silver amalgams and vaccinations contribute to mercury overload. Fish consumption has high mercury levels, especially in large fish, such as tuna. Heavy metals disrupt the immune system.

Toxic buildup occurs in the colon, liver, and kidney.

Breast cancer, which now affects one in every eight women in North America, has recently been linked to the accumulation of chlorine compounds in breast tissue. A study carried out in Hartford Connecticut, the first of its kind in North America, found that: "Women with breast cancer have *50% to 60% higher* levels of organochlorines (chlorination byproducts) in their breast tissue than women without breast cancer."

Needless to say then, that everyone must implement detoxifying into his or her health routines.

Naturopaths and Homeopaths treat toxicity, both physical and emotional with Bach Flower remedies, homeopathic remedies, herbs, and supplements.

Toxins

The word "toxin" is derived from *tox*, which means: poisonous.

Below are some facts about toxins:

- Toxins are substances, which are harmful to your bodies.
- Toxins can create free radicals, which cause damage to your cells.
- Toxins can destroy enzymes.
- Toxins can interact with hormones, creating imbalances in your glands.
- Exotoxins are toxins that come from outside the body: herbicides, pesticides, metals like lead or mercury, viruses, bacteria, parasites, caffeine, alcohol, meat, molds, pollens, EMFs, radiation, etc.
- Endo-Toxins come from within the body from intestinal bacteria and flora, acids, hormone overload, free radicals, toxic emotions, and memories.

Your body has several means at its disposal to deal with toxins. Your main detoxifying systems are:

- **Blood** – your blood carries nutrients and oxygen to all parts of your body and exports waste products to the lungs, liver, and kidneys for detoxification and elimination.
- **Digestive System** – your digestive system has the enzymes to break down substances, including cancer cells. It separates the "clean" from the "unclean".
- **Skin** – your skin releases toxins through sweating, or perspiration.
- **Lungs** – your lungs release toxic gases.
- **Spleen, lymphatic system, and thymus gland** – each of these has detoxifying tasks.

Therefore, you need to assist these systems to function optimally.

The Lymphatic System

The Lymphatic System is the body's sewage system. The lymphatic system is very important in the removal of toxins in the body. However, because it does not have a "motor" of its own, like the way blood is pumped directly by the heart, lymphatic stagnation in the lymph nodes can occur. Keeping your lymphatic system moving along is very important. To get it going, muscular contraction needs to occur.

The heart receives three liters of lymph daily. Lymph is rich in white blood cells to fight disease. The lymph system's "motor" is your breathing rate, which is higher when you exercise. Lymph fluid is cleansed in your lymph nodes and then returned to your bloodstream.

How to Improve Lymphatic Drainage

Lymph movement depends on muscle contraction, breathing, as well as manipulation at times. Follow these tips to optimize lymphatic drainage:

- Do not wear a restrictive bra or metal underwire as it obstructs the flow around the breast.
- Perform lymphatic massage, either self-massage or by a massage therapist.
- Exercise, specifically at least 10 minutes daily rebounding on a rebounder. Jumping on a rebounder greatly improves the circulation of lymphatic fluid. The motion gently massages the liver and colon, increases oxygenation, improves digestion and elimination, and Improves cardiovascular health. Rebounding 10 minutes has the aerobic effect equivalent to 40 minutes of tennis or 30 minutes of jogging!
- Do daily skin brushing and contrast showers (alternating hot and cold water in the shower).

Other Information about the Lymphatic System

Here are some other useful facts related to your lymphatic system:

- **Lymph Nodes (600 of them)** – These cleansing factories filter lymph and fight infection.
- **Lymph Vessels** – Lymph transport vessels move lymph fluid through the body and can easily get clogged.
- **Lymph Fluid** – Lymph fluid circulates the debris.
- **Spleen** – The spleen stores blood and filtrates it.
- **Tonsils** – The tonsils are lymphatic tissue masses that offer protection from bacteria in the mouth and throat.
- **Thymus** – This gland houses the T-lymphocytes, which are the part of the immune system that seek and destroy cancer cells. They coordinate the immune system's response to cancer.

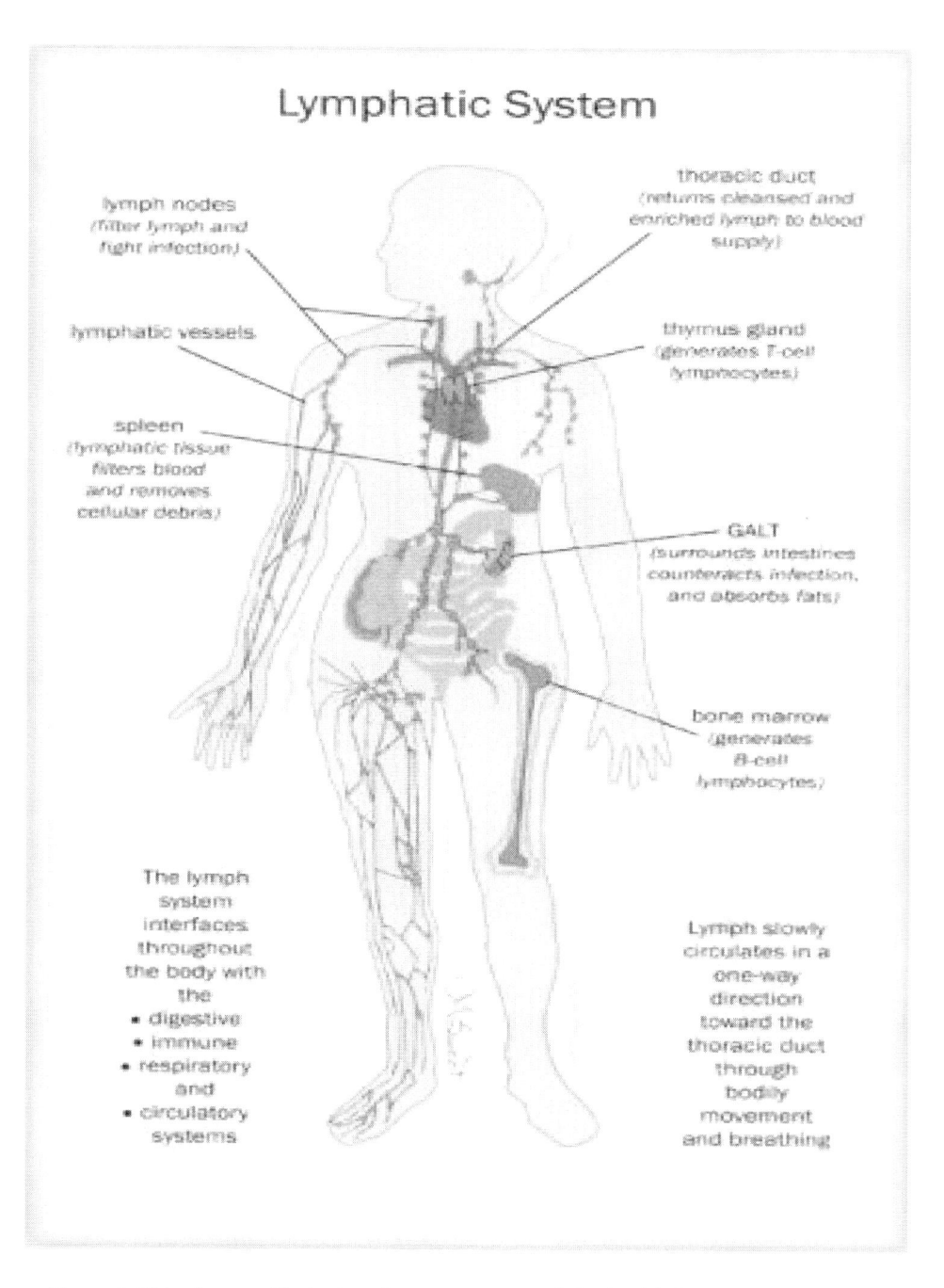

Figure 1: This diagram illustrates the components of the body's lymphatic system.

How to Detoxify

Here are different ways we can help our body's detoxification systems do their job:

Method	How the Body Detoxifies
Biological Dentistry	**Avoid Root Canals**! Dental toxicity: Nickel, chrome, zinc, iron, mercury, and cadmium are all used extensively in dental restorations. Many people do not realize that "silver" amalgam fillings are 50% mercury. A large filling may contain as much mercury as a thermometer. Mercury is the most toxic element on earth. Due to its poisonous nature, mercury can affect the whole body, including the immune system and digestive system, and affects your breast health. All these metals are found in breast cancer tissues. Some research studies have been found that a very high percentage of breast cancer patients had root canals or other infections on the same acupuncture meridian that runs through the breast. Ensure that you visit a biological dentist, who is trained to recognize the impact of toxic materials and specializes in the safe removal of amalgams.
Bowel Cleanse Colonics	Improve your bowel flora by taking a probiotic. Increase the frequency of bowel movements by the use of fiber and water. Examples of foods high fiber: Oat bran – psyllium husk – flaxseed. Consider colon hydrotherapy: removes waste from the large intestine. Waste is softened and loosened with pressure-regulated water into the colon and evacuated through natural peristalsis. Colonics remove toxins and parasites in the colon.
Herbs	Herbs promote detoxification. For example, milk thistle benefits the liver, spleen, kidneys, and digestion. Other useful herbs for detoxification include schizandra, dandelion root, bupleurum, globe artichoke, celandine, and barberry.
Kidney Cleanse	Improve kidney drainage by drinking more water. For a kidney cleanse, take a bunch of parsley or cilantro, or coriander Leaves: wash them; then cut them in small pieces and boil in water for 10 minutes. Let the liquid cool down, filter it, pour in a clean bottle, and keep it inside refrigerator. Drink one glass daily, and you will notice all salt and other accumulated poison coming out of your kidney by urination. You will notice a remarkable difference.
Liver Cleanse	Do a 10-day liver cleanse twice a year. Mix freshly squeezed organic orange, lemon and lime juice to make 1 cup. You can dilute this mixture. Add 1-2 cloves of fresh garlic plus a bit of fresh ginger juice or grated ginger. Mix 1 tbsp of extra virgin olive oil and blend all. Drink in the morning one hour before eating.
Minerals and Vitamins	Certain substances speed up the detoxification process: zinc, copper, magnesium, molybdenum, iron, calcium chorine, niacin, riboflavin, vitamins C, E, A, and B complex. Other nutritional supplements to speed phase I detoxification are I-3-C or DIM, B3 (niacin), B1, Vitamin C, fish and flax seed oil, and seaweed.
Sauna	Your skin is your biggest detoxifying organ. Ideally, you should sweat daily such as through exercise or sauna. The heat from an infrared sauna goes deep and is very effective. Did you know that a nutritionally supported sauna detoxification plan of approximately 150 hours could rid you of 90% of your lifetime-accumulated toxins?

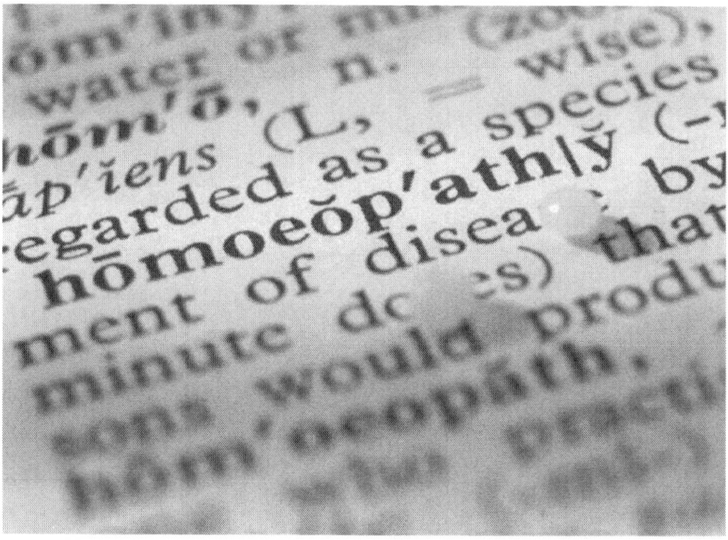

wise),
(L,
egarded as a species
hōmoeŏp'athy̆
by
ment of disea
minute

CHAPTER 7
THE ROLE OF EMOTIONS IN BREAST HEALTH

Most illnesses have both a physical as well as an emotional cause. There is a link between the amount and type of stress in your life and cancer.

In her book, *Heal Your Body: The Mental Causes for Physical Illness and the Metaphysical Way to Overcome Them*, Louise Hay describes the emotions associated with these physical elements:

- **Breast(s)** – Represent mothering, nurturing and nourishment
- **Breast Cysts, Lumps, Mastitis** – A refusal to nourish the self, putting everyone else first. Over-mothering, overprotection, overbearing attitudes
- **Cancer** – Deep hurt, long-standing resentment, deep secret or grief eating away at the self. Carrying hatreds. "What's the use?"

The Carcinogenic Personality

In homeopathy, we describe the carcinogenic personality as "other-centered" people. In other works, people who do things for others before they look after their own needs. Such people must learn to say, "NO."

Start to look after yourself before giving all to others.

The common emotional thread in cancer patients is unfulfilled passion that has been suppressed for many years. This pattern of suppression repeats itself over their lifetime. Oddly enough, studying piano later in life, or fulfilling another previously unfulfilled passion has an amazing transformational health effect.

In general terms, the carcinogenic personality profile can be summed up as follows:

- Loss/Grief (regarding relationship, status, etc.)
- Loss of a loved one
- Severe emotional stress
- Unfulfilled passion - Inability to be true to your own nature
- Unworthiness, hopelessness, or despair
- Avoidance of conflict - Fear of what others may think of you
- Tension in parental relationship

Homeopathy to the Rescue

I *love* homeopathy! I believe it is capable of actually *curing* disease instead of approaching the body as separate body parts and suppressing disease deeper within. Homeopathy takes the totality of the person, both physically and emotionally, into consideration ... *and that just makes so much sense! Doesn't it?*

It makes sense because you all intrinsically DO know deep inside that the body heals itself by getting rid of "stuff" (toxins). It makes good sense to look at the underlying issues instead of a short-sided approach of just looking at the symptoms. It just makes sense, if you just take a moment to really think about it, that a medical drug, which *is* a toxin, logically has to do more harm than good in the long run. How can something toxic to your body possibly heal you?

The public is simply so used to TV and radio advertisements about various drugs, even though nowadays, especially in the USA, they also provide a long list of side effects. How can that possibly result in cure or healing?

Homeopathic medicines have been around longer than pharmaceutical medications, which have really only been the system of choice since the American Revolution.

Research Study: Over 6,500 patients took part in a study at the Bristol Homeopathic Hospital. Published in the Journal of Alternative and Complementary Medicine on November 20, 2005, over 70% of patients with chronic diseases reported positive health changes after homeopathic treatment. A large variety of chronic diseases were included, such as eczema, asthma, migraines, irritable bowel syndrome, arthritis, menopause, depression, and chronic fatigue syndrome. The highest improvements were seen in children (89% of asthma patients and 68% of eczema patients under 16).

Homeopathic medicine promotes health and harmony of body, mind, and spirit through natural therapies. Through individualized treatment plans, homeopathic healthcare helps your body *heal itself* from illness. YOU are the only one who can do the healing for you, and we will educate and support you in this process. Your goals are to address the underlying causes of diseases, and to empower yourself in discovering what works best for you in healing and disease prevention.

Can Homeopathy Help Prevent or Treat Breast Cancer?

- Homeopathic medications have a wide range of use in treatment and prevention of breast disease.
- Homeopathy's goal in treating cancer patients is not only to cure, but also to prevent recurrence.
- Homeopathy searches for the trauma or trigger, which activated the dormant miasm (The word miasm means a cloud or fog in the being) or toxic influence.

Homeopathic Remedies for Radiation and Chemotherapy Exposure

Many remedies, such as hydrastis, thuja, iodium, conium, phytolacca, and asteria rubens are available to help the breast cancer patient chronically or acutely. See a classical homeopath specializing in homeopathic medicines to have your case taken.

Below are several homeopathic remedies used to treat those exposed to radiation or chemotherapy acutely:

- **Cadmium-Sulph** – Works as an antidote for radiation poisoning and relieves nausea. Relieves the intense gagging and retching after chemotherapy. It has a profound action on the stomach.
- **Radium Bromide** – Heals radiation burns that have resulted in ulcerations and severe aching pains all over.
- **X-Ray** – Boosts energy in patients with low vitality, chronic fatigue, and a sick feeling after chemotherapy and radiation. X-ray is indicated for mouth sores from treatment, anemia, and radiation dermatitis.

Other Ways to Protect Yourself from Radiation

Here are simple things you can do to help your body fight the effects of radiation:

- Include sea vegetables in your diet. Increase intake four-fold after exposure to radiation. Examples of sea vegetables are seaweed, algae, and kelp. Three kelp tablets per day is the recommended dose.
- Take turmeric, or curcumin. Note that it needs to be cooked with black pepper for absorption.
- Include flax oil in your diet to protect cell membranes.
- Drink green tea to remove radioactive isotopes. Steep the tea a minimum of 8 minutes.
- Eat miso soup, which helps your body excrete radioactive particles.

Imagery and Visualization: Yoga, Meditation, and Self Image

Did you realize that visualization could *alter* cellular mechanisms? What you imagine in your mind has a direct correlation to how your body responds to life.

Consider these examples from Jeanne Achterberg, author of the book, *Imagery in Healing*: *Shamanism and Modern Medicine*:

- A breast cancer patient shifts from being a "pleaser" or "victim" to doing what she always wanted to do.
- A woman describes that when she had breast cancer, she visualized little ghosts sweeping the cancer cells out with little golden broom.

Reference: www.jeanneachterberg.com

Yoga and Meditation – What They Offer

Yoga is a spiritual tradition, which seeks to bestow happiness and inner freedom rather than mere physical fitness and health. The word *yoga* in itself means joining; connecting the different levels of consciousness; spirit, soul, and body. With so many individuals now embarking on spiritual journeys, we need to honor the human spirit. In addition to basics, such as building self-esteem and a healthy ego, establishing boundaries and getting needs met, we need to go beyond ordinary consciousness, acknowledging the miracle of the *soul*, mystical experiences, and multi-dimensional awareness in therapy.

The Benefits of Developing a Healthy Self Image

Below are some benefits that stem from a healthy self-image:

- Becoming assertive
- Purging anger
- Resolving conflict
- Living with joy and purpose

Is It Possible to Prevent Cancer?

Yes it is possible. Not by swallowing pharmaceutical drugs and chemicals though. A safer alternative is looking at lifestyle changes. The American Cancer Society suggests you can reduce your risk of cancer by 62% with simple lifestyle changes.

Consider these:

- Reduce or eliminate processed foods, sugar, and grain carbohydrate intake.
- Eat organic foods when possible.
- Control your insulin levels.
- Balance omega-3 and omega-6 oils by supplementing with good quality oil.
- Get regular exercise (it drives your insulin levels down) and keep your body weight in control.
- Regulate your Vitamin D intake by getting plenty of sunlight exposure (Have a simple blood test at your doctor's office to get your levels checked).
- Get regular good sleep.
- Reduce your exposure to environmental toxins, such as in cleaning products and personal care products, as well as your exposure to pesticides
- Ensure adequate air quality.
- Limit your exposure to and provide protection for yourself from <u>information-carrying radio waves</u> produced by cell phone towers, base stations, phones and Wi-Fi stations.
- Avoid fried and charbroiled food; instead, eat a diet high in fiber.
- Work on your emotional health and balance. Even the CDC states that 85% of disease is caused by your emotions.
- Eat an 80% vegetarian diet with lots of raw food.
- STOP smoking!
- Detoxify the body on a regular basis, and reduce stress.
- Last, but not least, investigate safe screening techniques, such as Thermography and the estronex 2/16 urine test for breast cancer risk assessment.

THE FIVE "WHEELS" OF TOTAL HEALTH

I often compare caring for your body to caring for your car. It seems many of you take better care of your cars, than you do of your bodies. You make sure there is enough fuel, or energy, to run the car properly. You do regular oil, lube, and filter changes so that your car runs optimally. On weekends, you go to the car wash and polish your vehicles, clean the windows, and vacuum the interior.

What are the 5 "wheels" to take care of your bodies? What type of fuel, oil, lubes, and filters do your bodies need?

Wheel #1:		Water

Wheel #2:		Oxygen

Wheel #3:		Nutrients

Wheel #4:		Frequency - the earth's magnetic energy field

Wheel #5:		The steering wheel, represented by your *spirit*

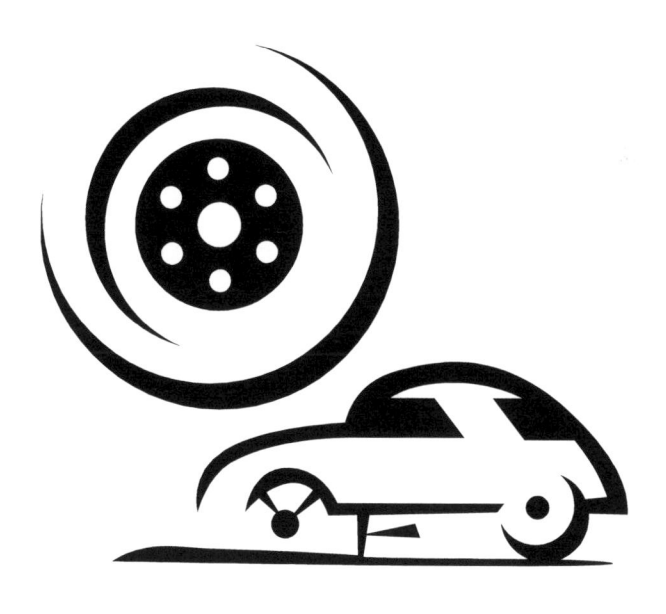

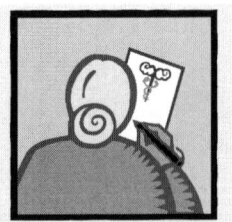

CHAPTER 8
YOUR COMPLETE 12-STEP ACTION PLAN

You have read a lot, and hopefully learned a few things. Now the hard thing is implementing new choices into your life. I like to take a "baby steps" approach and remind you that a new habit will take about six weeks to "take". It is true; practice makes perfect.

The baby steps may be different for everyone. I think for many, the most successful approach is to take 12 months to A New Healthy You, replacing not-so-good habits or downright bad habits with new ones.

You may want to consider working with a health coach to bring your intentions to completion. In a CNN interview, Dr. Mehmet Oz reported that health coaches should be a part of every public clinic, medical office, and hospital wellness center and that wellness coaches should be reimbursed by insurance companies and corporate wellness programs.

Carl C. Pfeiffer, MD, PhD
"For every drug that benefits a patient, there is a natural substance that can achieve the same effect." — Pfeiffer's Law

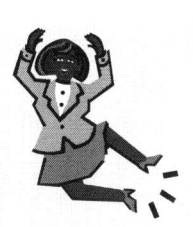

HOW TO HAVE HAPPY BREASTS

Start on your way to better breast health:

Exercise: Four hours a week can reduce your risk for breast cancer by 35-40%! Try rebounding exercises.

Stop Smoking

Nutrition:
- Vegetarian Diet: organic veggies – 5-8 servings a day. Eat more broccoli, cabbage, sprouts, kale, and collard greens (Brassicas). Eat more raw foods in general.
- Use unprocessed, organic olive oil and coconut oil.
- If you still eat meat, choose organic meats without hormones and antibiotics, and reduce your portions and the number of times a week you eat meat.
- Avoid <u>sugar,</u> as it depresses your immune system and feeds cancer cells.
- Eliminate milk and all dairy products. Dairy products contain both hormones and growth factors, in addition to fat and various chemical contaminants, which are implicated in the proliferation of human breast cancer cells.
- Strive for an 80% alkaline diet.

Supplementation: Take high-quality multivitamins and essential fatty acids.

Lymphatic Circulation: Do dry brushing, rebounding exercises to help eliminate toxins, lymphatic drainage massage, oils, etc.

Bras: Wear bras without underwire to allow more movement and, therefore, more movement of toxins out through the lymphatic system. Whenever possible and appropriate, go braless, and definitely sleep without a bra!

Breast Self-Exams: Still the best diagnostic test there is for detecting changes and lumps; 70% of all lumps are detected by women themselves.

Breast Self-Massage: There are wonderful breast oils and creams available and great combination aromatherapy oils which can be soothing and healthy to your breasts and your emotions.

Radiation: Avoid radiation exposure such as repeated X-rays (Yes, a mammogram is an x-ray!).

Baby Steps - Your 12-Step Action Plan

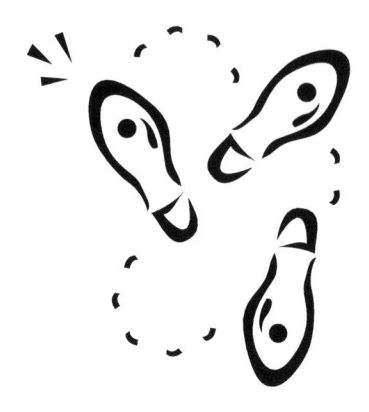

BABY STEPS (MONTH 1)

- ☐ **Water:** Let's start simply by looking at the basics you need in your life and those certainly start with <u>water</u> and <u>oxygen</u>.
- ☐ **Water:** Start each morning with a glass of water with lemon.
- ☐ **Breakfast:** Examine your breakfast, and add a few healthy things to it, or simply switch to make a healthy smoothie for breakfast, a wonderful start to the day. Add fresh ground flaxseed and flaxseed oil to your smoothie. You might want to take your vitamins at this same time. OR just add 2 tbsp of freshly ground flaxseed daily to your cereal, salad, or juice. Replace any sugary products with healthier choices, including fiber, and stevia as a sweetener.
- ☐ **Breathing:** Pay attention to proper breathing this month, or join a Yoga and Meditation group that teaches proper breathing exercises and techniques. Implement 10 minutes of breathing exercises before going to sleep, as it will help you to relax, balance your hormones, and detoxify.
- ☐ **Breast Self-Examination:** This first month, I would like you to do a Breast Self-Exam. Go to www.mammacare.com. Now set aside one time each month to do this breast self-exam. If you are still menstruating, choose a time five days after you finish your cycle. Hang a calendar in your bathroom to remind you, or place a sticky note on your mirror.

BABY STEPS (MONTH 2)

- **Water:** How are you doing with your water intake? Are you consistently drinking one a glass of water with lemon in the morning? If so, now add a glass of water at each of your meals and snack times. Review your breathing exercises and implement them if you have not done so.
- **Exercise:** Time to think about <u>exercise</u>. If you already go to a club or do any type of sport, you are good to go. Exercise about 40 min. each day if you can for a minimum of four days per week. Research getting a *rebounder*, as 10 min. a day on a rebounder is wonderful for your lymphatic system.
- **Lunch:** Now that you have a healthy routine for breakfast, let's examine your lunch and see how you can improve on what you are doing. Minimize meat and dairy, and add vegetables and fruits. Beans are a great option for wonderful salads. Try chickpeas, lentils, mung beans, kidney beans, etc. Add some nuts and seeds as your snack. Your goal is to get to 8 servings of fruits and veggies each day and/or use a green powdered supplement. Remember the Brassica family: kale, cauliflower, broccoli, broccoli sprouts, and cabbage preferably <u>raw</u>. If you are brave, start sprouting, and add these to your lunches.
- **Water pH Testing:** This month I would like you to test the water you are drinking and see what the pH is. If low, research a filtered water system, which will give you a high pH. Ensure you drink your water out of glass rather than plastics to avoid leaking chemicals that can affect your estrogen levels.
- **Fiber:** Add more fiber to your diet this month, and ensure you keep up the high water intake. Your goal is 45 grams of fiber daily.

BABY STEPS (MONTH 3)

<u>Review</u> how you are doing with the baby steps from Months 1 and 2. If you have not done or implemented some of these, use Month 3 to do those.

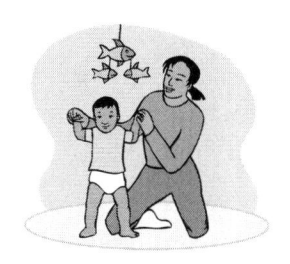

BABY STEPS (MONTH 4)

- **Plastics:** Let's look at the use of plastics in your house. As you might now realize, plastics, PVCs etc. are toxic and full of harmful chemicals. What plastic items do you have in your kitchen and your home? Research and buy alternatives to plastic, such as metal lunch containers for your kids, paper cups and plates instead of Styrofoam, glass containers instead of plastic storage containers, and cardboard or wood alternatives. Stop using plastic shopping bags. What else can you think of?
- **Dinner:** So are you doing pretty well with breakfast and lunch now? Time to look at dinner. That is often the hardest meal. You are so used to how you cook your dinners. First thing to consider is buying organic, especially fruits, vegetables, and chicken, if you eat it. Reduce your meat intake to only twice per week. Cut out dairy. Replace cow's milk with almond milk, and aim for an 80% vegetarian diet. I understand this is a lot of change for most, so again, baby steps. Where can you start this month? Pick one thing, and do it. Next month pick another thing. One year from now, you will have made 12 changes to your overall diet. That is huge. Suggestion: Instead of "cooking" tonight, make a plate of raw veggies and a homemade, healthy dip. Add some hummus and whole-wheat pita bread.
- **Turmeric:** Because of its properties to arrest cancer cells, add turmeric to your cooking each day, and use lots of garlic and onions. Use fresh rosemary, which is known to neutralize carcinogens.
- **Supplements:** The "fuel" for your bodies is nutrients, which are difficult to get completely from your diet even when you eat organic and raw. A good multi-supplement is important, and depending on your circumstances, health history, and drug depletions, you might need more that a multi-vitamin. I suggest reading or ordering the NutriSearch Comparative Guide to Nutritional Supplements, a compendium of over 1,500 products available and tested in the USA and Canada (www.nutrisearch.ca). Choose some good supplements for yourself this month, including a high quality fish oil or flaxseed oil supplement. If you can't eat eight servings of fresh fruits and veggies each day, buy a green powdered supplement.
- **Breast Thermography:** It is imperative to monitor your hormones and breast tissue health to stay in charge of your health. This month research and book a breast thermography appointment. (Go to www.thermographyclinic.com for a location).

BABY STEPS (MONTH 5)

- **Toxic Cleaning Products:** If you now understand that the toxicity build-up in your body plays havoc with your hormones and creates disease and cancer; you need to look at your personal toxic load and exposure. First, know that your skin is your largest organ, and everything you touch or put on it will be absorbed into your body. Let's start with looking at all the cleaning products you have or use in your house, from your dish detergent to the soaps you use, from the Windex to the bleach, and replace them with natural or green alternatives. Or simply make your own with basics, such as vinegar, baking soda, and borax.
- **Dinner – Part II:** How are you doing with making changes to your dinner? Make a list of the changes you have made, and be proud of yourself. Now choose something else you can add, subtract, or change this month. Look at incorporating more *alkaline* products in your diet. Go online and Google "alkaline food charts" to help you with this. A note about fish: Eating fish might sound healthier; however, the oceans and waterways are full of hormones, chemicals, mercury, and much more. Lots of mercury is present, especially in the big fish, such as large tuna, which are higher up the food chain, so avoid large fish and canned tuna, and stick with smaller species. Choose white meat over red. Research the fish you buy and where it came from.
- **Sea Vegetables:** Japan and China have a much, much lower incidence of breast cancer. Why is this? Definitely these countries have environmental pollution as we do, if not more. I think it is their diet, which boasts low meat consumption, no dairy consumption, and more sea vegetables. Incorporate seaweed or kelp into your diet. Experiment this month with eating a seaweed salad, or research a kelp supplement to add to your daily regime or smoothie.
- **Hormone Testing:** It is time to have your hormones tested. This month, ask your doctor to test you for: estrogen, progesterone, testosterone, free testosterone, DHEAS, LH, FSH; and for the thyroid: TSH, free T4 and free T3. From a naturopath or homeopath, have a saliva hormone test done as this test checks your bio-available supply of hormones: estradiol, progesterone, testosterone, DHEAS, and cortisol levels.

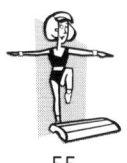

BABY STEPS (MONTH 6)

<u>Review</u> how you are doing with the baby steps from Months 1 to 5. If you have not done or implemented some of the suggested changes, use Month 6 to do those or fine-tune them. Pay specific attention to anything you skipped, and spend some time to understand *why* you did not do them before now. Look for the real emotions behind the initial response.

BABY STEPS (MONTH 7)

- ☐ **Toxic Cosmetics:** An area often overlooked is the toxicity of your cosmetics and your personal products. This month look at the labels of all your skin creams, facial products, shower products, shampoo and conditioner, soaps and make-up. Do some research online at the Campaign for Safe Cosmetics: <u>www.safecosmetics.org</u>. Realize there is bleach in your sanitary napkins and find a safer product to use against your skin.
- ☐ **Sauna Detoxification:** Did you know that 90% of your *lifelong* toxic load could be addressed with a well-designed, 150-hour (1 year), infrared sauna program? It is all about sweating it out. Sauna and sweating are great tools for eliminating environmental chemicals and toxic metals stored in your fat cells. However, sauna detoxification is not for everyone, especially those with conditions, such as lymphatic inflammation or heart disease.
- ☐ **Iodine Testing and Supplementation:** Last month, you looked at adding sea vegetables into your diet. This is a great way of upping your iodine levels, which is so important, not only for your thyroid and breast tissue, but also for your brain. Proper iodine levels help protect against the effects of estrogen. **Note**: Do not supplement with iodine if you have a <u>hyper</u>active thyroid. If you work with a naturopath, you can discuss iodine testing this month. Kelp is safe to use within your diet or as a supplement. Iodine can be found in sea salt, fish, asparagus, and spinach.
- ☐ **Yoga/Meditation:** Now let's give some attention to the mind, soul, and spirit because they need taking care of too. Toxic thinking or habits can be part of your physical ill health manifestations and **must** be dealt with. Traditional yoga and meditation practices are excellent tools to help deal not only with stress, but these practices may help with physical conditions as well and lower high blood pressure. Interview three yoga and meditation teachers this month, or find a video you can implement into your daily routine. Learning to do the Sun Salutation and proper breathing techniques can be both great fun and form very healthy habits.

BABY STEPS (MONTH 8)

- **Dinner – Part III:** It's now time to look at your progress in preparing healthy and nutritious dinners. Are you getting close to eating 80% vegetarian meals? Have you switched to mostly organic foods? Have you added 2 tsp of turmeric to your food daily? It is often not easy to eat 8-10 servings of organic fruits and vegetables daily. *Cooking tip*: Use extra-virgin olive oil for cooking. For frying, start with some water, and then add some olive oil. Another good option to use organic coconut oil. One final issue to tackle is your use of sugar. This month, I would like you to replace your regular sugar use with stevia, and if you have not already done so, <u>absolutely no consumption of soft drinks</u>! Drink organic green tea daily instead of soft drinks or coffee. You can make a nice ice tea with the use of stevia. Consider making your own lemon juice for your children with fresh organic lemons, filtered water, and stevia.
- **GMOs:** Avoid buying *genetically modified foods*. The most likely products to be GMOs are: soybeans, corn, canola, sugar beets, cotton, dairy, sugar, papayas, zucchini, popcorn, and ingredients hidden in baked goods. *Buy food labeled 100% <u>organic</u>*. The US and Canadian governments do not allow manufacturers to label something 100% organic if that food has been genetically modified or if that animal has been fed genetically modified feed.
- **Garden Pesticides:** Let's look at your garden this month and the products you use in it. Stop the use of pesticides on your lawns and in your gardens.
- **Colonics:** An excellent way to clean the colon is colon hydrotherapy, preferably at a clinic that uses the "Angel of Water" system, which is gentle and non-invasive. Find a clinic near you that offers this service, and book an appointment. If that is not possible, do an herbal digestive cleanse.
- **pH Testing:** Go to your pharmacy, and buy some pH strips or tape, or you can buy either of these online at Amazon. Go to the chapter in this book about how to test your pH levels, and see where you are.

BABY STEPS (MONTH 9)

Review how you are doing with the baby steps from Month 1 to 8. Look how much you have changed so far this year by taking baby steps! If you have not done or implemented some of the suggested changes, use month 9 to do those or fine-tune them. Pay specific attention to anything you skipped, and spend some time to understand *why* you did not do them. Look for the real emotions behind the initial response.

BABY STEPS (MONTH 10)

- **Sun and Sleep:** This month you will work on some basics. Exposure to sun – 15 minutes each day gives you your natural *free* supplementation of vitamin D, and sun exposure is the best way to receive it. Sleep – you need to ensure that you get enough restful sleep, as it is at night, when your bodies enter the "rest and repair" mode in which healing takes place. So respect your sleep! Do 10 minutes of deep breathing to relax, and balance your hormones before going to sleep. Ensure that you sleep in a dark, *dark* room, and to protect the melatonin production that takes place in the dark, avoid turning on the light when getting up and going to the bathroom as the light interrupts and stops this process. Furthermore, minimize the use of electrical items in your bedroom, and if you do have some, keep them at least three to four feet away from where you sleep. This suggestion includes your alarm clock and cell phone!
- **Liver Cleansing:** Now that you cleansed your colon two months ago, you can go ahead with a natural, liver cleanse or an herbal cleanse. I recommend the 10-day liver cleanse used by Dr. Sat Dharam Kaur in her book, *The Complete Natural Medicine Guide to Breast Cancer*, page 146. For this cleanse, she uses freshly squeezed organic orange, lemon, and lime juice to make 1 cup of liquid. She suggests adding 1-2 cloves of fresh garlic plus some ginger, mixing in 1 tbsp of extra-virgin olive oil and drinking this mixture each morning one hour before breakfast.
- **Weight Control:** I hope that going through all the lifestyle changes you've implemented over the last 9 months have possibly resulted in some weight loss, or that you have maintained a healthy weight. If you feel that you have some weight to lose, let's focus a bit on that by looking at your exercise program and your diet. Are you doing at least 40 minutes of exercise every day, like walking, swimming, dancing, or rebounding? Look at your diet, and see if perhaps you are overdoing it somewhere. Look at your intake of carbohydrates, sugar, or any detrimental snacking habits. It's time to say *good-bye* to those habits. Seek help to lose weight if you need to.

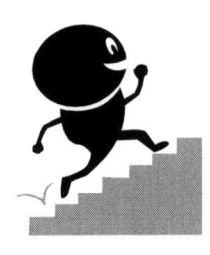

BABY STEPS (MONTH 11)

- **Canned Foods:** Last but not least in the Food Department of your life, lets look at your use of canned foods. As much as possible <u>avoid</u> the use of canned foods. Instead, look for things like tomato sauce or paste in glass containers. Many cans have plastic liners, which contain bisphenol-A (BPA), a nasty chemical affecting your hormones. In Canada, Eden Organic is an example of a safe company, which has BPA-free cans. Look for BPA-free labels on products, including bottles, baby bottles, children's drinking cups, and lunch boxes.
- **Dental Toxicity:** Dental toxicity is a big issue for many, who have still silver amalgam fillings, which contain <u>mercury</u>. When you do your next breast thermography, consider adding the Cranial/Dental/Thyroid Panel to see if you have any hidden inflammation. This month, find a biological dentist, and set-up a consultation. (http://iaomt.org)
- **80/20 Organic Vegetarian Diet Goal:** Time to have reached your 80-20% vegetarian and organic diet goal. Congratulations if you have, as *Food is Your Best Preventative and Healing Medicine*.

BABY STEPS MONTH 12

Eleven months of making baby steps in your lifestyle. CONGRATULATIONS! Time to celebrate and enjoy your new life and routines!

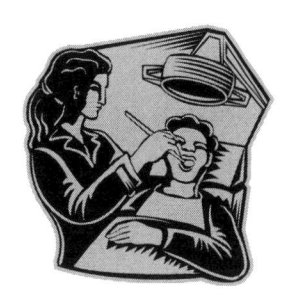

Personal Checklist:

I drink a glass of water with lemon in the morning.	
I drink 6-8 glasses of clean water each day.	
I make a breakfast smoothie and add flaxseed and oil plus vitamins.	
I eat a healthy lunch.	
I have tested my drinking water, checked the pH, and found a better option.	
I now eat 80% vegetarian.	
I now buy 80% organic foods.	
I consciously avoid GMO foods and buy 100% organic products.	
I eat many raw vegetables and fruits or take a green supplement.	
I eat 45 grams of fiber in my daily diet.	
I add 2 tsp of turmeric to my daily dinner.	
I frequently use healthy herbs, like rosemary.	
I only use olive oil and coconut oil.	
I added sea vegetables, like seaweed, to my diet or use a kelp supplement.	
I have replaced sugar with stevia.	
I no longer drink soft drinks or coffee and have replaced them with green tea.	
I do 10 minutes of deep breathing daily or before going to bed.	
I have learned helpful breathing exercises through yoga and meditation.	
I exercise 40 minutes each day and use a rebounder.	
I take daily multivitamins of a good brand, and flax or fish oil.	
I joined a yoga and/or meditation class.	
I now do monthly breast exams.	
I now do annual breast thermography.	
I no longer wear underwire bras.	
I do check my "Sexy Hormones" annually via blood and/or saliva testing.	
I have done some sauna detoxification or bought a personal infrared sauna for home use.	
I have done a series of colonics or an herbal digestive detoxification program.	
I have done my annual 10-day liver cleanse.	
I have visited a biological dentist and plan to remove my silver amalgam fillings.	
I have checked my iodine levels.	
I have replaced all plastic containers in my household with glass or stainless steel.	
I have replaced all toxic household cleaning products with green products.	
I have replaced all toxic personal care products and cosmetics with green products.	
I have improved my sleeping area.	
I have replaced all toxic garden products with green non-toxic products.	
I avoid buying canned products unless they are BPA free.	

12-Month Calendar: Action List

MONTH 1	MONTH 2	MONTH 3
Water Oxygen/Breathing Breakfast Breast Self-Exam No Underwire Bra	Water Exercise Lunch pH Water Test Fiber Intake	Review Months 1 and 2, and start the ones not yet done this month. ☺
MONTH 4	**MONTH 5**	**MONTH 6**
Plastics Dinner Add turmeric Supplements Breast Thermography	Toxic cleaning products Dinner - Part II Sea Vegetables Hormone Testing	Review Months 1-5, and start the ones you did not yet implement. ☺
MONTH 7	**MONTH 8**	**MONTH 9**
Toxic Cosmetics Sauna Detoxification Iodine Testing and Supplementation Yoga/Meditation	Dinner - Part III Garden Pesticides Colonics pH testing GMO	Review Months 1-8, and start the ones you did not yet implement or have stopped. ☺
MONTH 10	**MONTH 11**	**MONTH 12**
Sun and Sleep Liver Cleansing Weight Control	Canned Foods Dental Toxicity 80/20 Organic Vegetarian Diet Goal	Eleven months of taking baby steps and changing your lifestyle. CONGRATULATIONS! Time to celebrate. Enjoy your new life and routines!

REFERENCES and RESOURCES

PRINT RESOURCES and RECOMMENDED READING

Achterberg, Ph.D., Dr. Jeanne "Imagery & Healing: Shamanism and Modern Medicine' This influential book shows how the systematic use of mental imagery can have a positive influence on the course of disease and can help patients to cope with pain.

Armstrong, Liz, Dauncey, Guy and Wordworth, Anne "CANCER: 101 solutions to a preventable epidemic" This book offers solid evidence that many cancers are preventable, since their causes lie with the contamination of our bodies by pollution from the air we breathe, the products we use, the water we drink, and the food we eat. It is not being caused by just diet, smoking, and the noon-day sun!

Balch, Phyllis A., CNC and Balch, James F, M.D., "Prescription for Nutritional Healing" America's #1 guide to natural health - a practical A-to-Z reference to drug-free remedies using vitamins, minerals, herbs and food supplements.

Bathmanghelicij, F. M.D. "You're not sick, you're thirsty!" WATER for health, for healing, for life.

Beliveau, Richard Ph.D. and Gingras, Denis, Ph.D., "Foods to fight cancer: Essential foods to help prevent cancer" Detailing the key foods that have been medically shown to be beneficial in both preventing and fighting cancer, this is the must-have resource for anyone looking to get healthy and stay that way.

Campbell, Colin T. PhD & Thomas M. Campbell II "The China Study" The most comprehensive study of nutrition ever conducted. Startling implications for diet, weight loss and long-term health.

Clement, Brian R., PhD., NMD, LN and Clement, Anna Maria, PhD., NMD, LN "Killer Clothes" A book about how seemingly innocent clothing choices endanger your health and how to protect yourself.

Clement, Brian R., PhD., NMD, LN "Killer Fish" How eating aquatic life endangers your health.

Clement, Brian R., PhD., NMD, LN "Supplements Exposed" The truth they don't want you to know about vitamins, minerals, and their effects on your health.

Derry, MD, PhD., Dr. David "Breast Cancer and Iodine" How to prevent and how to survive breast cancer.

De Schepper, Luc, M.D., Ph.D., C.Hom., D.I.Hom., Lic.Ac "Hahnemann Revisited" A textbook of Classical Homeopathy for the professional.

Francis, Raymond, M.Sc. with Kester Cotton "Never be sick again" and "Never fear cancer again" Health is a choice Learn how to choose it.

Janzen, Jan "Breast Health Exposed!" 21 secrets most doctors will never tell you about your breasts.

Kaur, Sat Dharam, ND. "The Complete Natural Medicine Guide to Breast Cancer" A practical manual for understanding prevention & care.

Krop, Jozef J., MD, FAAEM "Healing the Planet one patient at a time" A primer in environmental medicine.
Lee, John R, MD "What Your Doctor may not tell you about Breast Cancer" How hormone balance can help save your life.
Meyerowitz, Steve "Power Juices Super Drinks" Quick, delicious recipes to prevent and reverse disease.
Vanderhaeghe, Lorna R., MS & Alvin Pettle, MD "Sexy Hormones" This book offers simple honest advice on how our hormones keep us young, enhance our passions and maintain our youth.
Vanderhaeghe, Lorna R., MS "An A-Z Woman's Guide to Vibrant Health" Prevent and treat the top 25 Female Health Conditions.

ON-LINE RESOURCES

www.breasthealthclinic.com
www.breasthealthexposed.com
www.centerforfoodsafety.org GMOs
www.cog.ca Canadian Organic Growers
www.drluc.com
www.drmercola.com
www.HealthierEating.org
www.mammacare.com
www.mammalive.net
www.thepassiontest.com
http://depts.washington.edu on Informed Consent
http://www.cancer.gov/cancertopics/factsheet/detection/mammograms For FACTS on Mammograms by the National Cancer Institute
Homeopathic treatment for chronic disease: a 6-year, university-hospital outpatient observational study. Dr. D.S. Spence, Dr. E.A. Thompson and S.J. Barron (Pub Med: http://www.ncbi.nlm.nih.gov/pubmed/16296912

Connect with Me Online

Facebook: http://www.facebook.com/breasthealthclinic
Twitter: http://twitter.com/breastclinic
LinkedIn: http://linkedin.com/in/cynthiasimmons
My blog: http://www.breasthealthclinic.com/blog
My e-book: www.HealthyHormonesGuide.com